LM

THE ULTIMATE
SOUP
CLEANSE

While every effort has been made to ensure that the information in this book is correct, it should not be substituted for medical advice. If you are concerned about any aspect of your health, speak to your GP. People under medical supervision should not come off their medication without speaking to their healthcare professional.

THE ULTIMATE SOUP CLEANSE

NICOLE PISANI & KATE ADAMS

First published in Great Britain in 2015
by Orion Publishing Group Ltd
Carmelite House, 50 Victoria Embankment
London EC4Y 0DZ
An Hachette UK Company

10 9 8 7 6 5 4 3 2 1

A CIP catalogue record for this book is available from the British Library.

ISBN: 978 1 4091 6491 3

Typeset by Us Now
Photography by Regula Ysewijn
Cover photography by Andrew Hayes-Watkins
Nutritional expert: Victoria Wells

Printed and bound by CPI Group (UK) Ltd, Croydon, CR0 4YY

The Orion Publishing Group's policy is to use papers that are natural,
renewable and recyclable products and made from wood grown in
sustainable forests. The logging and manufacturing processes are expected
to conform to the environmental regulations of the country of origin.

www.orionbooks.co.uk

For more delicious recipes, features, videos and
exclusives from Orion's cookery writers, and to
sign up for our 'Recipe of the Week' email visit
bybookorbycook.co.uk

CONTENTS

7. CLEANSE-ENHANCING RECIPES

8. BEYOND THE CLEANSE

CHAPTER 1: INTRODUCTION

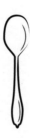

We'll be honest: however much we would like to be those people who treat their bodies as temples for 365 days of the year, the truth is that every now and then we need to balance out the inevitable indulgences with a few days of saintliness. The signs are clear when our trousers feel tight and somehow we always seem to feel hungry, fancying every cake or pastry that we see.

Our bodies get used to eating and wanting more rather too quickly – that it doesn't seem to happen the other way round very often seems to us to be one of life's cruel little ironies. But if we can gather our collective willpower and fill our cupboards with delicious ingredients for making quick and easy healthy recipes that we actually enjoy eating, then we give ourselves the best chance for getting off to a fresh new start.

In working hard the past five years to keep off the weight she lost all that time ago, Kate has found that it is much easier when she focuses on the things she can eat, rather than worrying about all the things she can't. We don't think extreme deprivation works; we believe that nourishing works, which is why you'll discover appetising, healthy, joyful soups that we hope will become your favourites of the future. For us, food is always an adventure and should also be a source of enjoyment.

Treat yourself to *The Ultimate Soup Cleanse* to reset your inner and outer balance. Feel good, eat well and enjoy:

- Losing weight

- Waking up with energy

- Feeling less bloated

- A better night's sleep

- Less stress

- Feeling clearheaded

- Falling back in love with your body

Our philosophy is very simple: to eat a wide variety of natural, healthy and seasonal foods and to cook them all from scratch. Eating and living this way even feels indulgent and like a treat, as we take the time to shop for interesting ingredients, plan recipes and enjoy every mouthful. We become more aware of our tastebuds and how we're feeling. We try our best to think before we eat, look for ways to be more active and also take the stress and over-complication out of life.

It might not happen all at once; it's often a good idea to make one small, realistic change at a time and to use that as a catalyst to make other sorts of tweaks and improvements. We kid ourselves that there are people out there who are somehow perfect in every way – they never eat chocolate; they do meditation and yoga every morning before the rest of us are even awake and putting the kettle on. Perfection is highly overrated, because in reality it's impossible and living that way would probably be pretty boring. We are all imperfect, but wonderful as we are.

It's often tempting to think that we need to completely overhaul our lifestyles, to become the 'new me', and put aside all the positive things that we do already in our lives. We are great believers that one change can lead to another, and that we can feel good all the way along the journey. Even when it comes to eating a little less or a bit more healthily, we need to get used to how different our body feels when we're not grabbing food whenever we feel like it but, rather, making conscious choices about what we eat. There's a lovely Buddhist saying that rather than feeling that small good deeds don't make a difference, one should imagine a jug that fills 'drop by drop'.

We have therefore designed this soup cleanse in such a way that you can start simply with a 2-day cleanse over a weekend or, if you'd like to commit for longer, we have a variety of 5- and 7-day cleanses. We hope the recipes offer inspiration as much as guidance and that they are a catalyst for falling in love with the healthy side of you, the one that might even like kale and tofu (we promise!).

1. RESOLVE

2-day ultimate cleanse to resolve any excess
water retention and give your body a break.

2. REBALANCE

7-day weight-loss cleanse.

3. RESTORE

7-day cleanse for restoring and
strengthening digestion.

4. RENEW

5-day nutrient-rich energising cleanse.

CHAPTER 2:
WHY CLEANSE?

For us, a cleanse is simply a way to bring ourselves back into balance. You know that feeling when you have been overindulging for too long, or you wish you could get up in the morning with a little more of a spring in your step and generally just feel more energised? Or there are the times when we know our digestive system is struggling – we might feel bloated or sluggish, or perhaps intolerant to foods that when we're on holiday or feeling great we can enjoy with no problems.

When we're willing to listen, our bodies give us all the signs we need to know that a few days of simple eating and living are a good idea. In today's fast-paced world, it's not always easy to slow down; many of us tend to get away with constantly running on empty, with the odd holiday here and there to just top up our reserves. Taking the time to restore and replenish and look after your body feels like a luxury that is out of our reach, but when you do give yourself this gift, the benefits will last.

SIGNS THAT YOU MIGHT BENEFIT FROM A CLEANSE:

- Decreased energy

- Feeling tired after eating

- Suffering from constipation, loose stools or irregular bowel movements

- Having a foggy brain

- Having trouble sleeping or finding it hard to wake up

- Feeling anxious or stressed lots of the time

- Having cravings for specific foods or feeling a dependence on certain foods

- Feeling bloated

- Experiencing weight gain

- Feeling generally 'off' your game

WHAT A CLEANSE AIMS FOR:

- A renewed sense of vitality and clarity

- Support towards achieving a sustained healthy weight

- Promoting deep and restorative sleep

- Regular, healthy bowel movements

- Energy throughout the day

- Positive, balanced relationship with food

- Feeling revitalised and enthusiastic about life

WHY GO ON A
SOUP CLEANSE?

*'The transformation which occurs in the cauldron is
quintessential and wondrous, subtle and delicate.'*
I Yin (239BC)

Soup came into being about five millennia ago when humans began to farm and cultivate food in addition to hunting and gathering it, and this marked a crucial stage in their development. When people began to put different ingredients into a pot with water over the heat of the fire, they created broths, gruel and stews. Before this, food had always been either roasted, fried or baked separately. The discovery of boiling and simmering foods together meant that a much greater variety of plants and grains could be combined and added to the diet, and meat could provide even more nutrition when the bones were boiled.

These bone broths were served in the first restaurants, which appeared in Paris in the eighteenth century. These *restoratifs* were usually meat consommés or bouillons that would help to 'restore' a person's strength and vitality: hence the word 'restaurant'. Bone-based broths have been used for centuries and across cultures as healing remedies, and chicken soup is worthy of a book of its own. Soup has long been used as a tool in various traditional medicines. In Ayurveda, a soup *(kitchari)* cleanse is undertaken to help restore your digestive 'fire', which is not only related to how our body digests the food we eat but also all our thoughts and emotions. Stoking this fire, or *agni*, is a way of supporting our overall health.

In Chinese medicine, it has been thought for thousands of years that consuming a bowl of soup before each meal is beneficial to one's health, and now research also suggests that this practice leads to eating fewer calories on average over the course of the day.

So soup is not just restorative, it's a great choice if you want to lose weight healthily. The good news is, you don't have to stick to that infamous cabbage soup, which according to our best Googling attempts no-one ever actually claimed to inventing. In fact, when it comes to eating well, variety has been shown to be a crucial factor for making positive long-term changes and choices. We enjoy a food trend as much as anyone – our cupboards are filled with coconut oil, kale and various seeds that we're not quite sure what to do with – but we also love the simplicity and the heritage of soup. It is restoring; it's clean and comforting. It also turns out that soup has even more than the test of time on its side when it comes to weight-loss benefits.

Soup has been shown by researchers to keep us fuller for longer per calorie compared with eating the same foods 'dry'. This is because in soup form the foods take up more room in the stomach, which turns off the appetite or 'hunger' hormone quicker than a salad would. Ghrelin, the hunger hormone in question, is released by specialised cells in the stomach wall when the stomach is empty. The hormone then travels via the bloodstream to the brain's appetite centre, the hypothalamus, to tell you that you are hungry. When your stomach is full, ghrelin is no longer released and so the appetite signal is switched off. Soup takes longer to leave the stomach, which is why you stay satisfied for longer. In an experiment conducted by the BBC programme *10 Things You Need To Know About Losing Weight,* the participants who ate soup reported feelings of fullness for up to an hour and a half longer than the control group eating solid foods with a glass of water.

WHY COOKING IS SO GOOD FOR YOU

When you cook from scratch, you tend to eat more natural foods that have undergone less processing. You also know exactly what you are putting into your body and so you are more aware of how certain foods make you feel. Despite scientists' best efforts, there really is no one-size-fits-all approach when it comes to knowing which diet is best for an individual. Some people are absolutely fine with dairy, for example, while others don't feel so great. Wheat isn't the evil enemy it's made out to be: for lots of us, it's the industrial process by which bread is now baked in order to reduce its preparation time that makes us bloat or causes a stomach ache. When we bake our own bread, using a variety of flours rather than just wheat, we make the wonderful discovery that we don't have to go through life without bread or pastries.

A key to keeping up healthy habits beyond just a few days is to be adventurous and explore new foods and ways of cooking. Nicole has recently become obsessed with sea spaghetti (seaweed shaped like spaghetti). She will use it alongside noodles, in salads, to liven up lentils – and more. It just so happens to be wonderfully good for you, too.

We find the art of preparing food to take care of your inner temple is soul replenishing. Feeling good about treating yourself well, to present your food to yourself with those little touches, such as toasted nuts and seeds or a drizzle of herb-infused oil, makes the cleanse a pleasure rather than a sacrifice. Sit down to eat, take time out of your day to be mindful of what you are eating and how you are feeling. We hope that this way it will be possible to enjoy the journey equally as much as the end result.

EAT NATURAL

Bircher Muesli takes its name from Dr Maximilian Bircher-Benner, who was a Swiss physician and pioneer in nutritional research. In 1904, Dr Bircher-Benner set up a sanatorium called 'Vital Force', which was based on the German lifestyle reform movement that espoused the idea of living in harmony with nature. Instead of the usual diet of meat and potatoes, Bircher-Benner recommended eating more fruit, vegetables and nuts.

The more we can live with an awareness of nature, the better it is for our bodies, too. This is what the healthiest cultures in the world have been doing for thousands of years; the Mediterranean diet is based on what's available and grown in the region – olive oil, fish and vegetables; while for the people of Okinawa it's fish and seaweed, and for the Koreans it is kimchi – a traditional dish made from fermented vegetables and spices.

The people of these cultures eat what is naturally available to them and we feel equally passionate about all the amazing foods grown in our own countries – for Kate that's the UK and for Nicole it's the island of Malta. In the UK, it feels as if we have traditionally been a land of hunters and gatherers, what with all the berries, game, fish, wild mushrooms, nuts and herbs that proliferate. Malta is an island of sunshine, a land with ripe tomatoes, figs, olives, fish and an incredible sourdough-type bread. We have an abundance of foods available to us year round, and as soon as you tap into choosing as many unprocessed foods as possible, you begin to really notice and experience the vibrancy and vitality of seasonal produce. There is an organic vegetable farm near where Kate's parents live, about two hours from London and whenever she gets to visit she returns with a bag full of the brightest, crispest vegetables which are still dusted with glistening drops of dew from when they were picked or pulled that very morning. All these ingredients are full of flavour and cook almost instantly because they are so fresh. If you can find food like this, you can't really go wrong.

EAT WITH THE SEASONS

Nature has a way of providing us with foods that are particularly good for us at certain times of the year. During the autumn and winter months there are plenty of ingredients that are perfect for warming soups and stews: carrots, squash, sweet potatoes, parsnips and so on, then in the spring, when our bodies are feeling stronger, nutrient-rich leafy greens are to be found in abundance, and in the summer, when we need cooling foods, there are cucumbers and lettuces. If you eat what is seasonally available in your own country and climate, you will naturally eat much of what your body needs at a particular time.

AUTUMN/WINTER CLEANSING

Autumn and winter are not when our bodies instinctively want to cleanse, but with so many of us enjoying the holiday season and all the treats on offer, it is a time when we often feel a need to balance out our over-indulgences. We tend to feel more hungry in cold weather, and we do need to keep warm and take care of our immune system, so going on a 100 per cent raw food diet at this time might be a little more than our already strained digestion can handle. This is why soup is such a great way to cleanse; it's the ideal solution for eating a little less, eating natural ingredients, and eating foods that nourish our digestion back to optimum health.

Tips for your autumn or winter cleanse:

- Keep warm – take baths and wear plenty of natural cotton or wool layers, and thick socks or slippers in the evening.

- Stick to warming foods like soup rather than ice-cold juices. If you enjoy a raw salad, balance it with a warm soup first or enjoy fermented vegetables such as kimchi (pages 141 and 184) or sauerkraut.

- Drink plenty of herbal teas.
- Create a mood board for the New Year (see page 19).

SPRING/SUMMER CLEANSING

We don't think it's a coincidence that the spring is a time of deep cleaning on all fronts – from the house to our diets, to life in general. In the winter we need to conserve our energy, and in the spring that energy can be harnessed and put into action as the days become a little warmer and lighter and signs of life appear all around us in nature. Many of the green shoots that begin to grow during spring are perfect ingredients for clean eating – such as nettle tops, dandelion greens and pea shoots. Summer is naturally a time to enjoy ourselves, so early summer is a great time for a cleanse ahead of dancing away the midsummer nights.

Tips for spring/summer cleansing:

- Think green in the spring and add vibrant greens to your meals wherever possible.
- Depending on how your digestion feels, i.e. if it is feeling strong, you can add raw garnishes to your soups, such as sprouted seeds, grated carrots and shaved fennel.
- Get outside as much as you can to take advantage of the increasing levels of natural light.
- Sow seeds to crop later in the year – either in your garden, or just in a window box or in pots on a windowsill.
- In the summer your body naturally needs a little less energy from food, which is the perfect trigger to go for lighter choices and recipes.
- This is a great time to enjoy chilled soups.

Quite often, when we think of eating healthily we think of having to cut out all the things we like and to try our best to stay on a diet for as long as possible before desperation or boredom gets the better of us. We hope that the ideas and recipes within these pages will prove to you that healthy food can make us feel really good and can inspire us. Kate is always telling Nicole that she could open a health-food restaurant if she wanted to because her recipes never taste like 'diet food', just delicious. This is the key to a happy and healthy relationship with what we eat and how we feel about ourselves and our bodies. Love food, love your body.

MIND AND BODY WORKING TOGETHER

'Tell me what you eat, and I will tell you who you are.'
Brillat-Savarin

We need to be willing to listen to and sometimes talk to ourselves when we are on the road to making healthier choices because our body and mind aren't always in unison, especially to start with, and with so many 'quick-fix' foods at our fingertips every day the temptations never really go away.

Mindfulness is a strong ally when it comes to changing our eating and living habits. It is easy to let days to go by in a blur, as we get through what we need to do on autopilot and look forward to that moment at the end of a busy day when we can sit down for a couple of minutes. We often forget to have breakfast, grabbing lunch absent-mindedly, thinking more about what we're going to do next rather than what we're doing right now. Often, we spend our time looking forward to those few days of relaxation that we have on holiday each year, counting down the weeks to when we can finally put our feet up, only to then put pressure on ourselves to have the perfect holiday!

When you begin to cultivate mindfulness, you bring a little more calm and relaxation into everyday life while at the same time being more observant about how you feel at any moment, noticing what and how you are eating and giving yourself a bit of space before making choices. At the end of a hard day's work, your body will all too easily rely on old habits for finding comfort, whether your habit happens to be ordering a pizza or having a glass of wine. All mindfulness does is allow you to observe those habits and the feelings or triggers attached to them so that you can then ask yourself what it is that you really need in order to feel good, to sleep well and wake up energised.

Mindfulness also encourages us to slow down while we are eating and instead of grabbing something on the run and hardly noticing what we are eating as we gulp it down, to switch off external distractions (yes, smartphones) and concentrate on our meal, enjoying each mouthful. When you respect food in this way, just for the few minutes it takes to have a meal, you respect your body and the relationship between the two. It may sound a bit fanciful, but mindfulness is now prescribed on the NHS to alleviate depression, stress and anxiety disorders.

Brian Wansink from Cornell University has conducted various studies on the relationship between our minds and our eating habits. In one, he was interested to find out what triggered people to stop eating, and so he created a special soup bowl which could be continuously refilled via an invisible tube. A table was half laid out with bottomless bowls and half with normal bowls and the participants were invited to sit down to eat and chat together over 20 minutes. They were then asked to give their opinions about the soup to the researchers. In just 20 minutes, those participants with a bottomless bowl had consumed an average of 75 per cent more soup than those with regular bowls. This suggested that a major trigger that tells us to stop eating is when we have finished the food on our plate, rather than an awareness of how much we have actually eaten. So if we can keep an eye on the size of our portions, we have a good chance of improving our eating habits while enjoying our food at the same time.

CONSCIOUS CLEANSING

■ You will notice quite a bit of variety in our soup cleanse recipes. This is partly because Nicole is a chef and loves the challenge of creating recipes that are delicious, healthy and don't leave you feeling hungry, but it's also because variety keeps you mindful about what you are eating. We could easily tell you to eat the same two soups every day for a week and you'd soon lose weight. The problem is that you won't have changed any long-term habits and you won't have had to think about what you're eating throughout the cleanse. With a variety of ingredients and choices, you're taking your own diet and way of living into your own hands. As a result, it will become more obvious how your body feels after eating certain foods, and what your body wants in order to feel really good.

■ Before you eat, take a few moments to use your senses to appreciate your meal. Breathe in the aromas of the food, take in its appearance with your eyes. As you cook, enjoy the rhythm of chopping and stirring, bringing ingredients and flavours together.

■ Writing things down always helps to make them stick in our minds and our habits. It may be as simple as writing a food and exercise diary of everything we have eaten and how many steps we have taken during the day; this kind of awareness feeds our motivation. A mood or vision board is also a great way to visualise a healthier lifestyle, with gorgeous photos of ingredients and recipes and places we'd like to go. This kind of gentle monitoring and checking in has been shown to really help with changing habits for the long term.

■ Don't leave healthy habits entirely at the mercy of your willpower, as it's a finite resource that is easily used up, particularly by the usual stressful events that we need to tackle on a daily basis. Being prepared is one of the best ways to help your willpower; the fewer temptations you have in your cupboards at home and the more delicious and healthy foods you have on hand, the better. Don't put off lunch, and never eat at your computer; the more you savour your food the more nutrition you will absorb.

CHAPTER 3:
THE PRINCIPLES

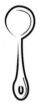

Neither of us is a dietitian or nutritionist, so we teamed up with Victoria Wells, who is a nutritionist and also a food lover. Victoria has offered us nutritional advice on maximising each cleanse. Nicole has a chef's instinct for balance in meals and Kate has worked with experts across a wide range of disciplines – from Dr David Servan-Schreiber, author of the acclaimed *Anticancer*, to fertility expert practitioner Emma Cannon and women's health expert Marilyn Glenville – always with a fascination for the relationship between how we feel and what we eat.

Different experts have different ideas about what exactly a 'cleanse' might be, but for us it's simply a chance to give ourselves and our bodies the opportunity to rest, restore and renew, to take a bit of time to help our often stressed digestive systems and help our bodies' natural detoxification processes.

We feel an instinctive leaning towards the individualised approaches of traditional medicines such as Chinese and Ayurveda, and in the more modern context we understand the potential benefits of visiting a nutritionist or clinic to help pinpoint one's own specific strengths and weaknesses when it comes to diet and digestion.

We also believe there is much we can do ourselves, in making choices that can improve how we feel, what we eat and our overall relationship with food. For example, Kate has always been relaxed about food, but when she is stressed her healthy habits go haywire and she feels the same emotions about food as about whatever is stressing her! She has discovered that to regain her healthy relationship with her body, and therefore build up her digestive 'fire' once again, she also needs to give herself a break and chill out.

Whatever science tells us, our own experience is equally one of our greatest teachers. Take coffee, for example – there are studies that will tell you it's good for you and others that advise to steer clear. The only person who really knows how coffee affects them is the individual. And it might change depending on how you are feeling generally, how busy you are or what kind of shape your digestion is in. On holiday a cup of coffee might be just what you fancy, but when you're working all hours and feeling low on energy you find yourself reaching for more and more cups to keep going while knowing that you're feeling overly wired at the same time. That's your body's way of telling you a caffeine cleanse is a good idea (and it really is surprising how quickly we lose the perceived need for coffee once it's out of our system).

It's the same for things like wheat and gluten. Only people with coeliac disease have a true gluten allergy and cannot tolerate it in any amount. For the rest of us, we need to decide for ourselves or with the help of a nutritionist if we feel better cutting out gluten or if it's more a case of not eating highly processed, mass-produced grains and instead opting for breads like rye, spelt and sourdough which are made using traditional methods.

A QUICK GUIDE TO THE DIGESTIVE SYSTEM

It is through digestion that our body breaks down food into nutrients and absorbs what it needs to survive and thrive. It is a combination of the organs of the digestive system along with hormones, nerves, bacteria and blood that perform the complex task of processing what we eat and drink each day. It is amazing what the digestive system will manage to cope with, but when we push things too far we soon begin to suffer the consequences and feel less than 100 per cent, both physically and in our mood.

The digestive system is made up of the digestive or gastrointestinal (GI) tract and the liver, pancreas and gallbladder. The GI tract begins with the mouth, then the oesophagus, stomach, small intestine and the large intestine to the anus.

Digestion begins in the mouth, as we chew our food and release saliva, which moistens the food and also releases an enzyme that begins to break down the starches in the food. This enzyme, lingual lipase, also starts the breakdown of fats in the mouth although the major breakdown occurs in the small intestine. Even the speed at which we eat and chew is thought to have an effect on our digestion – if we can slow down as we eat and chew our food more thoroughly we can make an instant, easy change for the benefit of the rest of our digestive system.

Once we swallow, the food passes through the oesophagus to the stomach, where it is mixed with stomach juices which contain an enzyme that breaks down the protein. The broken-down food is then released slowly from the stomach into the small intestine where it is mixed with juices from the pancreas that break down carbohydrates, fats and proteins, and with bile from the liver that dissolves fats. Bacteria in the small intestine also produce enzymes to help digest carbohydrates. It is thought that these bacteria in particular, our gut flora, are affected by modern diet and lifestyles, but equally we can have a positive effect on our gut health by eating fewer processed foods and opting for a variety of natural foods instead.

Digested nutrients are absorbed through the walls of the intestine into the bloodstream, which then carries those nutrients throughout the body. The waste products are pushed into the large intestine, where any water and still-remaining nutrients are absorbed and what's left is turned into stools to be stored in the rectum and then eliminated from the body in a bowel movement.

The body has hormones that regulate our appetite, signalling when we are hungry or full. We also have nerves that release chemicals to speed up or delay digestion.

KIDNEYS

The kidneys are not part of the digestive system but they are worth mentioning here as they are responsible for removing waste and extra water from the blood after your body has taken what it needs from the food you eat. Generally, a healthy diet rich in antioxidants is also beneficial to the kidneys, including cruciferous vegetables – for example, cabbage and cauliflower – and the allium family of garlic, onion and leek, along with berries, apples, oily fish and olive oil.

SIGNS OF
WEAKENED DIGESTION

When our digestive system is under too much pressure and begins to strain at the edges, there is a number of signs that can flag up that things aren't running as smoothly as when everything is in optimal working order. These include:

- Bloating
- Excess wind
- Constipation
- Heartburn and indigestion
- Loose stools
- Fatigue
- Headaches

When any symptom persists for longer than two weeks it's advisable to seek medical help. However, we wanted to give an outline of some of the common digestive system problems that many people experience at one time or another. There are entire books devoted to conditions like IBS and candida, so we can only really touch the surface here. It seems to us that these conditions are becoming increasingly common, but perhaps it is that we are more aware of them and want to address these kinds of health issues and improve our quality of life rather than continue to feel below par indefinitely.

BLOATING

Many women regularly experience the discomfort of bloating, particularly as the day goes on. It can be caused by overeating or eating too quickly, excess wind, constipation, candida overgrowth, water retention or food intolerance. As with many digestion issues, it's usually a case of narrowing down the potential causes. If you read 'eating too quickly' and think, 'oh, that's me', then it's easy to focus on eating more slowly for a while to see if it makes a difference. Likewise, if you know you don't like drinking water and probably only have a glass a day, try to find some herbal teas that you like to drink, or make naturally flavoured waters (page 177) to increase your water intake and see if that helps. Dandelion tea is a natural diuretic that can work wonders with water retention, and contains many nutrients and beneficial compounds, so it's great for a cleanse and just to enjoy as a drink every now and then.

Too many fizzy drinks can cause bloating and we steer clear of them on the cleanse. Also, it is thought that raw food can trigger bloating for some people, which is why we focus on foods that are generally considered to be more easily digestible and are cooked in ways that make them easier to digest, such as soups.

EXCESS WIND

Although adding more soluble fibre to your diet, such as fruit and vegetables, is generally a very good thing, one disadvantage is that it may cause you to suffer from increased gas. Of course, it is perfectly normal to produce gas, but it can be a problem if it becomes excessive or has a bad smell. A good probiotic can be helpful, to repopulate the gut with beneficial microbes. Try having a cup of chamomile tea after you eat, as it may help to relieve gas.

Excessive gas may be due to a mild but irritating food intolerance. Unfortunately, and especially if our digestive system is a little weakened, we can be intolerant to 'healthy' foods such as beans, broccoli, cauliflower, Brussels sprouts, leeks, garlic and onions. If you suspect this might be the case, the best way to find out is by first keeping a food diary to help pinpoint the potential culprits and to then try an exclusion diet, where you eliminate all the possible irritant foods and then introduce them again, one by one, noting how they make you feel. Generally, if you begin to ease up on your digestive system by not overloading it too much it will strengthen and might begin to become tolerant once again to foods that previously triggered bloating and gas. (See page 29 for more on food allergies and food intolerance.)

CONSTIPATION

A regular bowel movement can range from three times a day to three times a week: whatever is regular to the individual. Anything less than that, though, is considered constipation and can start to feel extremely uncomfortable. There is plenty of fibre included in the cleanses that follow, which alongside drinking plenty of water and herbal teas throughout the day should ensure good bowel movements. Soups are thought to be helpful, too, as is the avoidance of processed foods, and even giving ourselves the time to go to the toilet in a relaxed way rather than always in a rush.

LOOSE STOOLS

Long-term bowel irregularities should always be investigated by a doctor; this can rule out any infections or more serious conditions.

Loose stools may be triggered by stress and anxiety, or by specific foods. You can try eliminating these and then reintroducing them into your diet one at a time to see if one in particular is the specific cause. Common triggers are caffeine, dairy, highly-saturated fat food, such as red meat, and citrus fruit.

Kate has also found that taking a course of good probiotics alongside a little apple cider vinegar at mealtimes can help improve the gut flora and therefore digestion in general. A nutritionist can give tailored individual advice to your personal situation.

HEARTBURN AND INDIGESTION

Heartburn is when a little stomach acid goes up into the oesophagus, causing that burning sensation and chest tightness. Certain foods can make this worse, including fatty foods, alcohol, juices, chocolate and, for some people, onions and spices. Eating too much, too fast, can cause the acid reflux, as can being overweight, so eating healthily and mindfully is a good idea for preventing heartburn. Probiotics are thought to help, as are mint and chamomile teas.

FOOD ALLERGIES AND INTOLERANCE

As a chef, Nicole has noticed over her career the increasing numbers of customers with food allergies and intolerances, and so she understands the importance of being notified about a customer's allergy to nuts, shellfish or gluten, for example. However, she is less thrilled when alerted to an intolerance such as to tomatoes. Are more people becoming sensitive to dairy or gluten, or are we just more readily saying so now? Are we worrying too much about specific ingredients when it is in fact the way in which they are processed that's making us intolerant?

You can pick a side of the debate and you can always find evidence somewhere and somehow that will back you up. As food lovers, we opt for eating as much variety as possible, eating as little processed food as possible, and then trying to be aware of how foods make us feel as individuals. Kate finds peppers and cucumber skin 'unsettling', while too much cow's milk tends to trigger indigestion for Nicole. We're very lucky, we know, because it's not hard to avoid peppers and cucumber skin, but perhaps there is something to be said for an attitude towards food that means we are excited to try everything. We also realise that there are times when we instinctively feel the need to simplify our diet and have a bowl of rice and veggies. It's when we don't listen to our bodies that we tend to end up with a food hangover.

IRRITABLE BOWEL SYNDROME (IBS)

Although increasing numbers of people are reporting symptoms that are associated with IBS it is still a very difficult condition to diagnose, because there is not yet a specific test to say definitively if a person has it or not. To reach a diagnosis of IBS is often quite a long journey of excluding other possible conditions, including Crohn's. IBS is termed a syndrome because it is a collection of symptoms, all or some of which may be experienced to varying degrees.

Symptoms of IBS include:

- Diarrhoea
- Constipation
- Alternating diarrhoea and constipation
- Abdominal cramps
- Bloating
- Excess wind
- Nausea
- Indigestion
- Mucus in stools
- Fatigue
- Headaches
- Backaches
- Sleep disruption
- Period pains
- Painful sex for women
- Mood swings
- Anxiety
- Depression

Often anxiety can trigger the physical symptoms of IBS, while the onset of a physical symptom such as diarrhoea can in turn heighten anxiety, creating a negative cycle that is difficult to escape. Sufferers often feel both emotionally and physically exhausted, fearful of eating out and being constantly on alert.

Obviously these symptoms are quite wide ranging, which makes it difficult to pinpoint first that someone is suffering from IBS and then what is causing it, so that positive steps can be taken. The key issue is that bowel habit has significantly changed for a period of time.

Although the exact causes of IBS haven't been established, there is still much that individuals can do (especially with the help of a good nutritionist) to investigate possible causes and to begin to calm the symptoms through healthy eating habits – giving the gut a break from irritants, dealing with stress, and building a strong digestive system.

It is thought that some cases of IBS are triggered by a previous case of food poisoning or gastrointestinal infection. Some people are thought to have more sensitive nerves in the bowel, so they need to look at whether particular foods trigger spasms and pain. For others, it might be related to antibiotics disrupting the healthy gut flora. Hormones can have an impact on symptoms, as can yeast overgrowth (*Candida albicans*).

The cleanses in this book are not designed specifically to help with IBS, but simplifying your diet for a few days and taking time out to rest and relax can be helpful both for calming the gut and beginning to pinpoint if any specific foods are causing sensitivity.

We have a friend whose digestive system completely broke down due to an infection and she ended up in hospital for months. She could hardly eat anything that didn't trigger sensitivity and pain. But over time, she decided that rather than live this way for the rest of her life she would gradually build up her digestive fire enough to be able to increase the variety in her diet. She did such a good job that she now eats everything again in moderation. This isn't possible for everyone, of course, but it does show that sometimes there is a great deal we can do to help ourselves.

WHICH CLEANSE
IS RIGHT FOR YOU?

A cleanse doesn't 'detox' your body, the aim is simply to lighten the usual workload on your body's digestive system for a short period of time. If you provide your body with foods that are easier to digest and give yourself a break from the usual stresses and strains of daily life, you allow your body to rest and recuperate and build up some of its energy reserves once again.

For this book we have created four cleanses, each with specific goals in mind.

1. RESOLVE

This is a 2-day cleanse designed to resolve the problem of excess water retention and give your body a break from any foods that may be inflammatory. It is perfect for a quiet weekend when you want to balance out recent over-indulgences. It's also a great kick-start to a healthy weight-loss lifestyle change (particularly if you include the Rebalance cleanse), and an excellent reset for when you can just begin to feel yourself falling back into unhealthy habits. This cleanse is the perfect reminder for your body and mind of how great it feels to eat delicious, healthy food and take time to take care of yourself.

GOALS

■ 2–3lb weight loss (including excess water)

■ Banish excess bloat

■ Reset healthy habits

■ Take time out

2. REBALANCE

A 7-day weight-loss cleanse that begins with the Resolve kick-start weekend and continues in a more gentle way through the week with plenty of good fats and healthy protein to help retrain your appetite thermostat while eating a little less. It is possible to lose up to 7lb in this week – 4lb of which is likely to be excess water.

GOALS

- 5–7lb weight loss (including excess water)

- Keep on the move throughout the day

- Try something new every day

- Love food, love your body

3. RESTORE

This is a 7-day cleanse focused on restoring and strengthening digestion. As the brain and gut are connected, this is also a great way to improve mental concentration and focus. This cleanse lays healthy foundations for the long term; it includes not only restorative foods, such as bone broths and fermented foods, but also restorative exercise that is reconnecting and gently strengthening, stoking up your fire from within.

GOALS

- Relight digestive fire
- Improve gut flora
- Promote long-term healthy weight management
- Regain clarity and mental focus

4. RENEW

A 5-day, nutrient-rich, energising cleanse that is a great tune-up when you feel like you'd rather stay in bed and pull the covers over your head than go out for a run or cycle ride. Go for Renew when you'd like to get your joie de vivre back. It's always difficult to describe just what 'vitality' is, but somehow we just know when we feel we have it and, conversely, when we're not quite firing on all cylinders.

GOALS

- Replenish energy reserves
- Wake up with vitality
- Grab life with both hands

A HEALTHY WEIGHT FOR YOU

There is no 100 per cent foolproof way to know what your healthy weight is, but the Body Mass Index can be helpful because it indicates a healthy range.

Weight lb	100	105	110	115	120	125	130	135	140	145	150	155	160	165	170	175	180	185	190	195	200	205	210	215
Height	Underweight					Healthy						Overweight					Obese					Extremely obese		
5'0"	19	20	21	22	23	24	25	26	27	28	29	30	31	32	33	34	35	36	37	38	39	40	41	42
5'1"	18	19	20	21	22	23	24	25	26	27	28	29	30	31	32	33	34	35	36	36	37	38	39	40
5'2"	18	19	20	21	22	22	23	24	25	26	27	28	29	30	31	32	33	33	34	35	36	37	38	39
5'3"	17	18	19	20	21	22	23	24	24	25	26	27	28	29	30	31	32	33	34	35	36	36	37	38
5'4"	17	18	18	19	20	21	22	23	24	24	25	26	27	28	29	30	31	31	32	33	34	35	36	37
5'5"	16	17	18	19	20	20	21	22	23	24	25	25	26	27	28	29	30	30	31	32	33	34	35	35
5'6"	16	17	17	18	19	20	20	21	22	23	24	25	25	26	27	28	29	29	30	31	32	33	34	34
5'7"	15	16	17	17	18	19	20	20	21	22	23	24	25	25	26	27	28	29	29	30	31	32	33	34
5'8"	15	16	16	17	18	19	19	20	21	22	22	23	24	25	25	26	27	28	28	29	30	31	32	32
5'9"	14	15	16	17	17	18	19	20	20	21	22	22	23	24	25	25	26	27	28	28	29	30	31	32
5'10"	14	15	15	16	17	18	18	19	20	20	21	22	23	23	24	25	25	26	27	28	28	29	30	30
5"11"	14	14	15	16	16	17	18	18	19	20	21	21	22	23	23	24	25	25	26	27	28	28	29	30
6'0"	13	14	14	15	16	17	17	18	19	19	20	21	21	22	23	23	24	25	25	26	27	27	28	29
6'1"	13	13	14	15	15	16	17	17	18	19	19	20	21	21	22	23	23	24	25	25	26	27	27	28
6'2"	12	13	14	14	15	16	16	17	18	18	19	19	20	21	21	22	23	23	24	25	25	26	27	27
6'3"	12	13	13	14	15	15	16	16	17	18	18	19	20	20	21	21	22	23	23	24	25	25	26	26
6'4"	12	12	13	14	14	15	15	16	17	17	18	18	19	20	20	21	22	22	23	23	24	25	25	26

WAIST TO HIP RATIO

To calculate your waist to hip ratio you simply divide your waist measurement by your hip measurement. For women, ideally this number should be less than 0.8 and for men less than 0.95. The reason to check this is that it's an indication of whether you are carrying too much weight around your middle, which is thought to be more dangerous to your health than if you carry a bit of extra weight around your hips and bum area.

Q&A

Q. Will I get headaches on the cleanse?

A. You may get the odd headache as you cut out caffeine and sugar. It's surprising how quickly our bodies do get used to not having these stimulants though, so stoke up your willpower for the first two days and it will get progressively easier after that if you choose a longer cleanse.

Q. Is it possible to shrink your stomach?

A. No, your stomach remains the same size regardless of what you eat. However, you can retrain your appetite to be smaller, and of course during the holidays it's easy to get used to eating more. It really helps if you eat slowly and mindfully, with no distractions.

Q. What about 'nightshades'? Should I avoid them?

A. There are some nutrition experts who believe the family of 'nightshade' foods should be avoided. These are tomatoes, aubergines, potatoes, peppers (bell peppers, chilli peppers, paprika, cayenne, tomatillos). There is no research to suggest they are a problem for the vast majority of people, but if you feel you are sensitive to these then do talk to a nutritionist to find out more.

Q. How much weight can I expect to lose?

A. It usually depends how much retained water you lose. Some people will lose up to 7lb in the first week, 4lb of which is likely to be water and 2–3lb fat.

Q. What if I get constipated?

A. There is plenty of fibre included in the cleanse recipes, so you should be fine, but sometimes our digestive systems aren't keen on change, like when you go on holiday and nothing happens for the first few days. Try to stay relaxed about it – Kate's best home remedy to get things moving is a teaspoon of molasses.

Q. Should I take any supplements?

A. It's best to talk individually with a nutritionist about whether you would benefit from any specific supplements. We do take a quality probiotic supplement when our digestion feels weakened to help build up the beneficial bacteria.

Q. What about 'superfoods'?

A. 'Superfoods' are really a marketing gimmick; all natural fruits and vegetables are great for you and you're probably as likely to absorb as many nutrients from broccoli and kale as you are from spirulina. If you happen to like any so-called superfoods, then go for it.

Q. Should I see a doctor or nutritionist?

A. Seeing a registered dietitian or nutritionist can be very helpful if you suspect you may be suffering from a digestion condition or you need some tailored help with you diet. Googling various symptoms can bring up many more questions than answers and having a professional consider your whole health picture can be very helpful. These recipes should be used in combination with a healthy lifestyle. If you are concerned about any aspect of your health, be sure to consult your GP.

Q. What if I think I'm intolerant to foods on the cleanse?

A. We are all individuals when it comes to food and so please do feel free to tweak the cleanses if there are ingredients that don't agree with you. We have deliberately included a wide variety of foods and haven't wanted to be overly restrictive, for example including beans and pulses which some people find a little hard to digest. Use the recipes in this book to inspire your taste buds and see what you really fancy.

CHAPTER 4:
PREPARATIONS

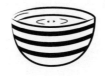

We often promise ourselves, 'tomorrow I'm going on a health kick', and then when tomorrow comes we find an empty fridge or, even worse, a bar of chocolate lurking in the cupboards and our healthy intentions quickly fly out of the window for another day.

The more prepared we are, the easier we find it to get back into our healthy habits. Get the spice cupboard fully stocked, fill the fridge with jars of vegetable and chicken stock, clear the kitchen work surfaces and pin your menu for the week somewhere in the kitchen where you can easily see it.

KITCHEN CLEANSE

Nicole definitely believes in the 'life-changing magic of tidying up' that Marie Kondo writes about in her bestselling book of the same name. A good tidy is something that brings benefits to all aspects of life, when you think about it. It's much easier to work on a clean desk, clear of clutter, with the one task at hand in front of us. Even our minds become full of clutter that we no longer need – old hurts and hang-ups, tensions and worries. Nicole loves to have clear surfaces and organised cupboards before she creates in the kitchen. And it really helps when preparing for a cleanse to have a good clear out of your cupboards so that you can look forward to stocking up and cooking some amazing recipes over the next few days.

SOUP EQUIPMENT

The good news about making soup is that it's much simpler to clean up afterwards than it is when you are juicing – all that pulp that just seems to stick to the equipment! Plus, that's the fibre, the good stuff, that we're throwing away. With souping, your best friend is your blender, followed by your Tupperware and flasks. You can make batches of soup on the weekend for the week ahead, so that all you need to do is heat them up and add a few nuts and seeds when you're ready to eat them. Easy.

Blenders

We have bought all kinds of blenders over the years and we find that the simple ones seem to work the best for us. A hand-held blender tends to mean less washing up, and if you have the patience to work out all the settings then a soup maker allows you to sauté your vegetables then add your stock and blend all in the same appliance. Nifty. There are also 'silent' blenders available if you can't stand the noise!

Flasks

We love the wide-brimmed flasks for soup. If you are able to heat up your soup at work during the day there are some great Tupperware soup containers available. Our favourite flask is the Black & Blum stainless-steel flask. It definitely makes soup look good.

STORAGE

Nicole tends to put everything she owns into Tupperware or jars. She has a cupboard very neatly stacked with just about every dimension of container you could think of. Nicole's best tip is to always try to find the size that leaves the least room for air at the top – that way your soup (or whatever you are storing) will last a bit longer. The vegetable and chicken soups are the easiest to store – best before two days.

STORE CUPBOARD ESSENTIALS

This looks like a long list but these are all ingredients that will keep well and will form the basis of a healthy, delicious store cupboard that you can fall back on any day of the week.

Olive oil

Coconut oil

Groundnut oil

Pumpkin seeds

Black and white sesame seeds

Flax seeds

Hemp seeds

Chia seeds

Almonds

Almond butter

Wheat-free (tamari) soy sauce

Ground or fresh turmeric

Cumin seeds

Fennel seeds

Mustard seeds

Caraway seeds

Cloves

Cinnamon

Cayenne

Nori flakes

Kombu (seaweed) sheets

Tamari wheat–free soy sauce

Brown miso paste

White miso paste

Dried or fresh shiitake mushrooms

Cider vinegar

Olives

Capers

Preserved lemons

Quinoa (including red or black if available)

Oats

Buckwheat

Brown rice

Wild rice

Brown rice noodles

Buckwheat noodles

Chickpeas

Mung beans

Aduki beans

Split peas

Red lentils

Puy lentils

Fennel tea

Dandelion tea

Green sencha tea

Raw honey

FRIENDS OF THE
SOUP CLEANSE

What are the key foods that will bring you the most nutrients? Well, it turns out that the best diet you can give your body is a varied one that includes whole foods such as vegetables, fruit, lean protein, whole grains, herbs and spices, legumes (beans and lentils), nuts and seeds, probiotics – for example, fermented foods such as kimchi and sauerkraut – and live cultures such as natural yoghurt and kefir. A combination of these foods provides a diet rich in antioxidants, fibre and pre- and probiotic foods that create the best environment for the good bacteria in our guts to flourish. This in turn means that we absorb nutrients from our food, release energy at a steady pace and waste is eliminated effectively.

ANTIOXIDANTS

Antioxidants are chemicals that interact with and neutralise free radicals or act as scavengers, helping to prevent cell damage, and are widely accepted by both conventional and alternative health practitioners to be beneficial for our health.

There are a whole range of good chemicals within the antioxidant family that are contained in a variety of foods:

- Vitamin C in berries and greens

- Vitamin E in vegetable oils, nuts and avocados

- Beta carotene in squash and carrots

- Copper in beans and lentils

- Manganese in nuts

- Lycopene in tomatoes

- Polyphenols in herbs

- Selenium in fish, meat and whole grains

- Allium sulphur compounds in garlic, onions and leeks

- Anthocyanins in aubergines

- Catechins in red wine and tea

- Flavonoids in green tea, citrus fruit and apples

- Indoles in cruciferous vegetables such as cabbage, cauliflower and broccoli

- Lutein in leafy greens and corn

- Zinc in seafood, lean meat and nuts

FIBRE FOR GUT HEALTH

Fibre is essential for our digestive health, which is why we've included plenty of fibre-rich ingredients in our recipes. Dietary fibre is an umbrella term used to group together the components of food that can't be digested and are therefore eliminated as waste in our bowel movements.

The two main forms of fibre are soluble – sources include oats, beans and fruits; and insoluble – which is found in whole wheat, nuts, seeds and some vegetables. The soluble fibre is broken down in the colon while the insoluble fibre remains mainly solid, although it is still fermented to a degree by bacteria in the digestive system. In his book *The Diet Myth,* Tim Spector assesses all the studies related to fibre (and many other food components) to try to understand why fibre does indeed seem like a good thing to include in our diet when it doesn't appear to do much except create waste. He discovered that the answer may lie in microbes, and in particular, prebiotics. Prebiotics act as fertilisers for our body's own microbes and allow good bacteria to thrive. All prebiotics are non-digestible fibres, and sources are listed on the next page.

- Asparagus

- Broccoli

- Dandelion greens

- Endive

- Garlic

- Jerusalem artichoke

- Leeks

- Onions

Other fibre-rich foods include:

- Avocado

- Barley

- Broccoli

- Chia seeds

- Flaxseeds

- Jerusalem artichokes

- Lentils

- Oats

- Peas

- Split peas

LENTILS AND PULSES

Some people find lentils and pulses quite hard to digest and may experience cramps, bloating and/or excess gas after eating them. We have some tips for making them more digestible:

- Soaking – instead of just soaking them in water overnight, soak them for 48 hours and change the water three times a day.

- Sprouting (pages 178–179) – sprouted beans are easier to digest.

- Slow-cooking – cook your lentils and pulses for as long as possible on the lowest heat.

- Kombu – put a strip of kombu seaweed in while soaking and also while cooking, then remove it before serving.

PROBIOTICS

The health of your microbes, or your 'gut flora' or 'good bacteria', in your digestive system appears to have a strong correlation both with digestive health and overall health and wellbeing. The good news is that both tradition and science offer us some easy and delicious ways to improve our gut flora.

Fermenting is an old-fashioned way of keeping food and it has recently seen a resurgence, both in the chef world and that of health promoters – it's nice when that happens. Foods like sauerkraut and kefir act in the same ways as probiotic supplements by improving your digestion health. The more friendly bacteria we can create in the world, the better.

Probiotic foods include:

- Kefir
- Kimchi
- Kombucha

- Live yoghurt
- Miso
- Sauerkraut

FASTING AND SNACKING

It is thought that giving your microbes a balance of work and rest is a good idea. We naturally do this when sleeping, but there is a growing school of thought that suggests that when we eat a healthy diet we don't need to worry so much about snacking to prevent blood sugar drops, cravings and feelings of irritability.

The trick is to get to know your own 'circadian rhythm', which basically means whether you are a morning or evening person. If you are an evening person, for example you find that you are alert and happy to work when most people have gone home for the day, you won't necessarily need to eat a huge breakfast. Likewise, if you do all your best work in the morning and find you would rather rest quietly in the evening, you don't need so much energy – in other words, food – later in the day. You may find that out of habit, boredom, or the need for a reward you eat every time you have a break, when really a cup of herbal tea would be fine until lunch or dinner.

This is something you can practise while on the cleanse, because you will become more mindful of how you really feel and what your body needs.

ANTI-INFLAMMATORY FOODS

Inflammation is specifically associated with conditions such as arthritis, chronic pain and gastrointestinal disorders including Crohn's and ulcerative colitis. A healthy diet that includes anti-inflammatory foods is not only of potential benefit to such conditions but also to our general health. Prevention is ev en better than cure, so if we can take steps to be aware of maintaining a healthy diet and lifestyle, we can help ourselves take care of our health. It is impossible to predict what health issues we may meet in our lifetimes, but being proactive without being obsessed seems like a good idea.

For centuries people all around the British Isles would dry seaweed to provide extra nutrition in the winter. Now we tend to think of Japan when we think of seaweed; the people of Okinawa are known for eating plenty of it, with residents living to the ripe old age of 100 and boasting healthy hearts and low cholesterol. Seaweeds contain energy-boosting B vitamins, which are good for the brain and skin and also strengthen the immune system. Nori is a rare vegetable that contains long-chain omega-3 fatty acids, which are particularly effective against inflammation.

- Turmeric is one of the most powerful natural anti-inflammatory ingredients known at present.

- Ginger root is also an anti-inflammatory and antioxidant.

- Seaweed is an underwater gem.

- Cold-water oily fish such as salmon, tuna, mackerel, sardines and anchovies contain anti-inflammatory omega-3 fatty acids.

- Antioxidant-rich fruit and veg (see above), particularly the carotenoids in carrots, sweet potatoes and squash, and the allium family of garlic, onion and leek.

- Monounsaturated fats found in olive oil, nuts and avocado.

NATURAL DIURETICS

There is a number of herbs and foods that are thought to help reduce water retention and/or bloating, and so we have included these in some of the recipes:

- Aduki beans
- Alfalfa
- Asparagus
- Barley
- Basil
- Buckwheat
- Caraway seeds
- Celery
- Corn
- Fennel
- Horseradish
- Kohlrabi
- Leek
- Lemon
- Mung bean
- Pea
- Radish
- Seaweed
- Squash
- Watercress

WHY WE PREFER ORGANIC, LOCAL AND SEASONAL FOOD

It isn't just choosing the food itself that matters when we make decisions about what we eat, it's also how it was grown, raised or produced and how far it had to travel to reach our table. Many people believe that organic food is just more expensive and there are no tangible benefits to buying it. However, we see organic food not only as a way to consume fewer toxins, but also to support a method of farming and producing that is more sustainable for the land and for the most part more ethical in the treatment of animals.

In the US, and increasingly in Europe and elsewhere, it is possible to know if the beef you are buying was grass-fed rather than being reared and kept in barns and fed only with corn. Likewise, the standards set by the UK's Soil Association for organic farmers and producers are reassuringly high. As far as the argument about organic foods being more expensive goes, we have discovered that in fact farm shops and farmers' markets often sell organic vegetables for less than the price of conventional veg in supermarkets. Organic meat is expensive but so it should be, and so we try to make it go a long way.

FOODS TO AVOID

These are divided into two groups. The first are foods that are probably best avoided whenever possible, except for celebrations and holidays – try to avoid these 80 per cent of the time. These include the majority of processed foods and also refined sugar. Then there are the foods which really depend on your own constitution, the context in which they are eaten and the amounts. For example, we are not against wheat or dairy, but we do understand that they are the kinds of foods that we can easily overeat and therefore become a little sensitive to. Some people are, of course, lactose intolerant and unable to digest dairy foods, but for the majority of us it is a case of finding the balance that feels right for us. We often find that once we give our digestion a little rest and recovery time we are then able to enjoy a wider range of foods once again without the digestive problems that we were previously experiencing.

PROCESSED FOODS

It's difficult to lump all processed foods into one 'bad' category, because some foods that are pretty good for us go through some form of processing to reach the shelf – foods like quinoa and buckwheat, for example.

The kind of processed foods we are talking about are all those aisles of biscuits, sweetened cereals, chocolate bars, crisps, pastries, processed meats (including most sausages and bacon), processed cheese, packaged bread and yoghurts with fruit syrups or any additives other than 'milk'. Many fast-food restaurants and takeaways offer highly processed foods, and however healthy they claim to be, most packaged snacks aren't all that natural when you begin to look closely at the label. And that's the key: check the ingredients of foods before you buy and if you're not sure about any of them, give them a miss.

SUGAR

Sugar has got such a bad name in recent years that many people have even begun to worry about eating fruit. However, it's not the naturally occurring sugar in fruit when eaten whole that is the problem, it's the ways in which refined sugar has crept into the average diet that is causing problems, and that does include fruit juices made from concentrate.

There is still a debate over whether sugar is now the predominant cause of obesity, but evidence to support this theory is beginning to stack up, especially when you consider the rise in children's obesity. Here in the UK, currently 10 per cent of children are obese when they start primary school, and by the time they leave primary school the figure doubles to 20 per cent. According to Rachel K. Johnson, lead author of a paper published in the American Heart Association (AHA) journal *Circulation*, too much sugar not only makes people fat, but also is a key culprit in diabetes, high blood pressure, heart disease and stroke.

Watch out for added sugar (includes 'sucrose', 'fructose', 'high fructose corn syrup') in:

- Baked goods

- Bread

- Breakfast bars

- Butter

- Cereal

- Fruit juice

- 'Fruity' water

- Jams

- 'Low-fat' foods – these will often have sugar added when the fat has been taken away

- Marinades

- Pizza

- Ready meals

- Salad dressings

- Sauces

- Yoghurt

ARTIFICIAL SWEETENERS

There is a whole host of artificial sweeteners now available, designed to help people consume less sugar. We prefer to avoid artificial or plant-derived but highly processsed sweeteners, instead opting for food that has gone through as little processing as possible. There is some evidence to suggest that choosing low-calorie options, in particular fizzy and soft drinks, does nothing to help people lose weight. Some nutrition experts say this can be explained by the theory that when we consume artificial sweeteners we are doing nothing to retrain our sweet tooth, and will therefore continue to crave calorific sweet foods such as cakes and biscuits. Artificial sweeteners may also alter your gut microbiome balance, so are best avoided.

Artificial sweeteners include:	Natural sweeteners include:
■ Acesulfame potassium	■ Agave nectar
■ Aspartame	■ Coconut or palm sugar
■ Mannitol	■ Molasses
■ Neotame	■ Raw honey
■ Saccharin	■ Raw maple syrup
■ Sorbitol	■ Stevia leaf extract
■ Sucralose	
■ Xylitol	

When you start looking into refined sugar and its natural alternatives, things can become a little confusing. Just a few years ago, agave nectar was hailed as the healthiest natural alternative to sugar available, until it was discovered to contain extremely high levels of fructose, much more than honey, for example.

Our own favourite natural sweeteners are raw honey and the less-processed coconut or palm sugar. 'Raw' honey doesn't go through the same processing and pasteurisation methods as regular honey and so retains more of the natural probiotics and enzymes. Honey contains a better balance of fructose and glucose than refined table sugar, so is more easily assimilated by the body. It is still best to eat it in small quantities, however, but a spoonful on your porridge is just fine.

ALCOHOL

Alcohol seems to us a bit like caffeine; when we're on holiday it's part of eating out and having fun, but when we're working hard it does nothing for our energy levels or alertness. If you do enjoy a glass of wine or three, especially over the holidays, then cutting out alcohol while on the cleanses gives you an immediate energy boost, especially in the morning, and you will likely find that you sleep much more soundly. Of course, alcohol is hard work for the liver, and not drinking is the best tonic you can give it, which is another reason to avoid it during the cleanses.

CAFFEINE

Caffeine isn't necessarily bad for you, but for the duration of the cleanses we suggest replacing it with herbal teas. Green tea does have a little caffeine in it, but it doesn't affect the body in the same way as coffee. Our aim in the cleanse is to bring ourselves back into balance and also improve our sleep patterns. Cutting down on caffeine is a helpful way to do that.

DAIRY

There are many unprocessed cheeses, as well as live yoghurt and kefir (also made with cow's milk) that contain lots of beneficial bacteria, which may be one of the reasons why the French diet is considered to be so healthy, despite at first glance looking as though it is full of all the wrong things: saturated fats in butter, milk, cheese and red meat, plus all that wine, croissants and bread. The thing is that most French people eat all of these foods in the right balance and amounts that are a natural part of their culture.

We have replaced cow's milk and butter during the cleanses with other natural ingredients, again to give the digestive system a break from what are quite rich foods. However, we are not against these foods generally and believe butter to be a food of the gods!

FOOD SWAPS

Try to swap butter for olive or nut oils (coconut, groundnut, sesame). As we've said, we are not anti-butter, as our philosophy is to eat and enjoy a wide variety of natural foods, but on the cleanse we have suggested substitutes for butter as it is harder to digest – plus olive oil in particular contains many health-giving properties. Olive oil is at the heart of the Mediterranean diet, considered to be one of the healthiest in the world. Many of the health benefits attributed to the Mediterranean diet are related to consuming olive oil, including helping to reduce the risk of heart disease and cancer.

Like butter, cream is high in saturated fat and so quite difficult to digest (we know that sinking feeling after a restaurant meal cooked with cream). We now prefer lighter, and also probiotic, options such as live natural yoghurt and kefir. We have also discovered that you can blend tofu into a vegetable soup for 'creaminess' (honestly!) while also adding protein.

We have also swapped cow's milk for nut, rice or soya milks: for the cleanse we have gone dairy-free – except for live natural yoghurt and kefir, which contain lots of beneficial bacteria. There are so many delicious and varied alternatives to cow's milk now, and our favourites are the nut milks: coconut, almond and hazelnut. Go for unsweetened varieties with no emulsifiers. We choose organic wherever possible because the farming methods used to produce them are usually less intensive.

WHEAT ... AND GLUTEN

Like so many people, we do generally try to eat fewer foods containing wheat, finding that when we consume too much bread, pizza and pasta we feel bloated and uncomfortable. That's the simple reason why we have made the cleanses wheat-free and instead have included more grains that are really grasses – such as quinoa, buckwheat and amaranth. We love rye bread (which is wheat free but does usually contain gluten) and when our digestion is good we enjoy sourdough.

Gluten seems to be another food enemy of choice right now. About 1 per cent of the population is thought to suffer from coeliac disease, which is an allergy to gluten and can only be alleviated by cutting out gluten entirely from the diet. In recent years, however, it is the rise of a newly named condition – 'non-coeliac gluten sensitivity' – that has grabbed the headlines and fed the expansion of the 'free-from' food industry.

The trouble is that the symptoms of any food intolerance are similar: bloating, cramps, excess wind and irregular bowel movements. The only way to really know which foods are the cause is to go on an exclusion or elimination diet. This is where you stop eating any of the potential trigger foods for 28 days and then re-introduce them one at a time to discover which you are sensitive to. This takes a huge commitment and it's easy to see why it might seem simpler to just cut out both wheat and gluten.

It may be that Nicole and I are just greedy food lovers at heart, but we're not keen on cutting out any whole foods and so we focus on the way ingredients are used and processed to keep our diet as varied as possible. We will therefore ban supermarket bread from our cupboards but will buy a loaf of sourdough from the local baker who mills their own flour. We have no scientific basis for it, but we also find no digestive issues with baguettes from the boulangerie in France or a starter portion of fresh pasta while in Italy. The old adage, 'when in Rome...' seems to work out pretty well for us, as food rules go.

Red meat

To give the digestive system a break from the usual workload, we do not include red meat during the cleanse. The only exception is bone broth in the Restore and Renew cleanses. We love the Chinese medicine approach to red meat, which is to think of it as a very rich food that is full of nutrients and therefore only needs to be enjoyed in small amounts. When you think of meat in this way, it makes sense to also look for the best-quality produce available, which for us means locally reared, grass-fed and organic.

ENHANCING THE CLEANSE

In this section we have included some ways in which you can enhance the effects of the cleanse. Eating natural foods will naturally benefit your skin from within. You may find your eyes become brighter, your skin more radiant and your hair and nails healthier. You can also take this time to try out other healthy rituals such as body brushing, oil pulling, salt baths and meditation.

Body brushing

Body or 'skin' brushing is something you can do at home every day to help stimulate your circulation. We excrete and eliminate waste products through our skin, just as our liver and kidneys are organs of elimination.

Skin brushing is also thought to support the lymph system that, like the bloodstream, goes all around our bodies, and is a major filtering system as well as helping us to fight infections as part of the immune system.

How to body brush:

Do this on dry skin for a couple of minutes before you shower:

- Use a natural bristled brush, ideally with a long handle so you can reach your back.

- Don't brush your face or anywhere that feels tender. Women shouldn't brush their breasts.

- Start gently.

- Always brush towards your heart.

- Start with the soles of your feet and then go up each leg.

- Brush from the hands along your arms to your shoulders.

- Brush upwards on the buttocks and lower back.

- Use a gentle motion on the tummy towards the centre.

- Brush from the back of the neck to the front and gently on the chest towards the heart (just to repeat – not on the breasts).

Note: if you have any medical condition, check with your doctor first.

Oil pulling

This is an oral and dental hygiene cleansing technique which has its origins in Ayurvedic medicine. It is said to draw out toxins, improving oral and dental health and apparently overall health, too. There are no scientific studies to support this theory, but anecdotally people report whiter teeth, cured hangovers and better breath.

How to do it:

- The practice involves gently swilling 1 teaspoon of cold-pressed oil (we use organic coconut oil) around the mouth for 20 minutes in the morning on an empty stomach. It doesn't have to be a vigorous action, just keep it gently moving around and make sure it reaches all the nooks and crannies of your mouth. The liquid does increase in volume as it mixes with your saliva, so only try a little to start with, and make sure you don't swallow any of it.

- After 20 minutes, spit out the liquid and rinse with some warm water and salt.

Epsom Salts Baths

Epsom salt is named after a saline spring at Epsom, in Surrey, and is a naturally occurring mineral compound of magnesium and sulfate. Studies have shown that these minerals are readily absorbed through the skin and may help with the elimination of toxins.

An Epsom salts bath a couple of times a week brings many benefits:

- Helps with inflammation

- Eases stress and relaxes the body

- Relieves aches and pains

- Improves the body's absorption of nutrients

- May help with constipation

Breathing exercise

This exercise simply gives your mind and body a few minutes of rest. In this breathing meditation, we use the breath so that the physical body may help to calm the mind and vice versa in a cycle of focused relaxation.

If you are able, find a space that feels light and open to you, as this will help your mind to feel open, too. Either sit on the floor or on a cushion, or simply sit with a straight back on a chair, with your feet comfortably resting on the ground about shoulder-width apart. Rest your hands in your lap in a comfortable position.

Check your posture, you should be sitting:

- Cross-legged

- Straight back (imagine a stack of coins)

- Shoulders stretched slightly outwards, like the wings of a bird

- Neck slightly bent

- Eyes open, focused slightly down about a metre in front of you

- Mouth slightly open with the tip of your tongue touching your upper palate

- Hands on lap, in a comfortable position

Now simply sit for a few moments and just be. Allow yourself to settle into your body and your position; let things become quiet.

Begin to focus on your breath, gently breathing in and breathing out. Don't hold your breath on the intake, just let it go out again at a pace that feels comfortable to you. Bring your mind to the breath – you might want to imagine tensions going out of your body on the out breath, or just focus on the rhythm of your inhaling and exhaling.

Your thoughts will still continue to rise up – don't worry too much about your mind wandering during this exercise, simply observe your thoughts as they appear, acknowledge them, then let them go, bringing your attention back to the breath.

Even focusing on the breath like this for just a few breaths before eating will immediately bring a sense of calm and may help to slow things down so you can eat mindfully and enjoy every bite. It is a great daily practice for relieving tension and letting the stresses of the day wash away.

Meditation on the body

In this simple meditation you allow your mind to take care of your body and bathe it in your appreciation. It's easiest to do this meditation lying down, with your eyes closed and your arms lying in a relaxed position by your sides.

Breathe gently in and out – just as you did in the first breathing exercise. Breathe from your belly and begin to sense all the places where your body is touching the bed or the floor – really feel those points of contact and allow yourself to sink downwards, feeling heavy and grounded.

Bring your focus back to the breath and the rise and fall of your stomach. Keep your attention there for a few moments before taking your mind on a journey around the body. You can start with your toes; imagine breathing positive energy or light in through the tips of your toes and through your feet. How are your feet feeling? Sense any tension and breathe with it, imagine your feet are completely relaxed.

Now come up your through your ankles to your calves and then your knees. Observe any feelings of tension or pain and continue to bathe your legs in positive energy. Bring your focus to all the different parts of your body; your hands, your chest, shoulders, back and neck, your face, your forehead and the crown of your head. Send your appreciation through your breath to all the far corners of your body and send love to any places of pain or tension.

You may also want to focus on your different organs and the amazing tasks they perform; your senses, too – being able to taste wonderful foods, see the world and listen to a friend. Whatever it is you are thankful for in your body, these are a few minutes in which you can observe and connect.

At the end of the meditation, bring your focus back to simply breathing in, and breathing out, back to your belly. Open your eyes slowly and have a stretch before calmly getting up.

This is an easy and very relaxing meditation to do while on any of the cleanses, as well as every so often in your daily life.

Cleansing is the perfect way to give yourself permission to take care of yourself, take a little time out and nourish your body and mind. It's like a reminder to ourselves that healthy eating and healthy living feel really good, that to wake up in the morning feeling refreshed is the perfect start to the day. It resets our sense of balance and we feel lighter all round. So let's get to them!

CHAPTER 5:
THE CLEANSES

RESOLVE

2-DAY ULTIMATE CLEANSE

GOALS

- ■ 2–3lb weight loss (including excess water)
- ■ Banish excess bloat
- ■ Reset healthy habits
- ■ Take time out

Put aside a quiet weekend for this two-day cleanse. Get plenty of rest and relaxation on both days, and treat yourself to essential-oil baths in the evening (our favourite is rose) and a mineral bath one evening (pages 64–65).

The ingredients in this cleanse will help to resolve any excess water retention, and are anti-inflammatory and gently nourishing. The soups are deliberately light, which is why this is just a two-day cleanse. It is designed to give your body a break from its usual workload, so give yourself a break at the same time and think of this cleanse as your own personal retreat. Read an absorbing book, go for gentle walks, or if you enjoy yoga, do some stretches and meditation.

Notes for the RESOLVE cleanse:

- Allow 12 hours between dinner and the breakfast the following day, this gives your digestion plenty of downtime.

- Combine calming activities such as reading, meditation or simply sitting in the sunshine with some gentle exercise such as walking and yoga.

- Drink cleansing teas during the day: green, fennel, dandelion.

- Skin brush (page 63) in the mornings.

- Switch off your computer for the weekend and any social media.

2-DAY RESOLVE MENU

Day 1

Lemon juice, mint and hot water
Miso breakfast broth (2 batches) (page 169)
Turmeric, ginger and lemongrass broth (2 batches) (page 190)
Leek, fennel and celery with red lentils (2 batches) (page 97)
Hot cucumber with salmon/barley (V) (page 95/96)

Day 2

Lemon juice, mint and hot water
Miso breakfast broth (page 169)
Turmeric, ginger and lemongrass broth (page 190)
Balti-spiced cauliflower (page 90)
Berry kefir booster (optional) (page 170)
Leek, fennel and celery with red lentils (page 97)

REBALANCE
7-DAY WEIGHT-LOSS CLEANSE

GOALS

- 5–7lb weight loss (including excess water)
- Keep on the move throughout the day
- Try something new every day
- Love food, love your body

This cleanse is designed to follow the Resolve Cleanse (which takes up the first two days) and continues for the remaining five days of the week with a menu that will help to banish any bloating or water retention and begin to burn fat. It will be different for each individual but you can expect to lose 3–7lb during the seven days. Meals throughout the week are light but sustaining, with plenty of lean protein, good fats and spices.

Our aim when we need to lose those holiday pounds is to recharge our desire for delicious healthy ingredients and also begin to reset our appetite. It's all too easy to fall into the habit of continual grazing and so we feel it's not actually a bad thing to begin to let ourselves feel hungry rather than instantly feed our seemingly bottomless appetite.

This is a week where it's so important to bring together the mind and the body. Sustained weight loss takes a firm commitment at the beginning, attention to and awareness of what and how we are eating and living as we lose the weight, and finding the healthy things we enjoy and can fall back on for the long term. Kate lost two and a half stone five years ago and has maintained that weight loss mainly by walking a great deal and never letting ready meals back into her life. And whenever she feels the need to get back into more healthy habits, she makes a big pot of kitchari.

Notes for the REBALANCE cleanse:

- On waking, drink hot water with lemon juice to awaken your body. Drink your favourite herbal teas throughout the day to help reduce any lingering water retention and stave off hunger.

- Keep active as much as possible. Walk whenever and wherever possible, and include at least 60 minutes of cardio exercise if you are able. Kettle bells, body pump, Zumba, spinning and CrossFit are all great choices.

- Try not to snack every mid-morning and afternoon, but if you really feel you may cave in to sweet cravings if you don't have a snack, eat a nourish bite (page 173). These are perfect for exercise days.

- Keep a food and mood diary through the week (and ideally beyond) to begin to be more aware of what you are eating and how foods affect your energy and mood.

- Find time to eat without the usual distractions of work or the television. Eat slowly and mindfully.

7-DAY REBALANCE MENU

Prepare ahead

Roast chicken (pages 187–8)
Chicken stock (pages 187–8)
Vegetable stock (page 192)
Seaweed broth (page 189)

Day 1

Lemon juice, mint and hot water
Miso breakfast broth (page 169)
Turmeric, ginger and lemongrass broth (page 190)
Leek, fennel and celery with red lentils (2 batches) (page 97)
Hot cucumber with salmon/barley (V) (pages 95/96)

Day 2

Lemon juice, mint and hot water
Miso breakfast broth (page 169)
Turmeric, ginger and lemongrass broth (page 190)
Balti-spiced cauliflower (page 90)
Berry kefir booster (page 170)
Leek, fennel and celery with red lentils (page 97)

Day 3

Lemon juice and hot water (with optional teaspoon of honey)
Overnight oats with yoghurt and apple (pages 166–7)
Seaweed broth or a cup of miso (page 189)
Courgette, lemon and thyme (2 batches) (page 107)
Coconut chicken with turmeric and kale/Sprouted soup (V)
(pages 106/140)

Day 4

Lemon juice and hot water

Overnight oats with nuts and berries (pages 166–7)

Lime and mint water

Courgette, lemon and thyme (page 107)

Sichuan pepper and chicken/Spinach and spiced onion (V) (pages 116/119)

Day 5

Lemon juice and hot water (page)

Miso breakfast broth (page 169)

Coconut water (page 177)

Lemon, chicken and mint with aduki beans/Five-spice tofu (V) (pages 112/108)

Turmeric, ginger and lemongrass broth (page 190)

Asparagus mimosa (page 104)

Day 6

Lemon juice and hot water

Overnight oats with nuts and berries (pages 166–7)

Avocado on rye

Horseradish and lemony squash (2 batches) (page 110)

Kitchari (with optional sautéed spinach) (page 111)

Day 7

Lemon juice and hot water (with optional teaspoon of honey)

Egg drop with nori (page 168)

Horseradish and lemony squash (page 110)

Turmeric, ginger and lemongrass broth (page 190)

Kitchari (with optional grilled prawns/Greek yoghurt) (V) (page 111)

RESTORE

7-DAY CLEANSE FOR RESTORING AND STRENGTHENING DIGESTION

GOALS

- Relight digestive fire
- Improve gut flora
- Promote long-term healthy weight management
- Regain clarity and mental focus

Your digestion is the key to your vitality and sense of wellbeing. You might eat all the nutrient-dense foods available but if you're not digesting them well, your body won't be able to absorb those nutrients. If you are experiencing a great deal of stress in your life, for example, all that stress will be putting pressure on your immune system and in turn potentially causing inflammation. You might develop food sensitivities or suffer from such symptoms as headaches, body aches and feeling tired all the time.

Symptoms associated with a weakened digestive system are becoming more widely felt by increasing numbers of otherwise healthy people. Blended soups are particularly good for nourishing and strengthening a weakened digestive system as the food is already warmed and has been partially broken down in the blender. This isn't to say that we don't also see the potential benefits of including raw food in the diet, but from personal experience we know that when our digestive system is in need of a little help, it's a good idea to eat more warming foods, especially later in the day.

Notes for the RESTORE cleanse:

- Eat slowly and without distractions.

- Take a probiotic to help your gut flora flourish and absorb more nutrients from the food you eat.

- Eat well in the morning and lighter in the evenings. Don't overeat.

- Eat fresh, seasonal and ideally local produce.

- Add raw foods later in the week as your digestion feels strengthened.

- Take moderate exercise and practise deep breathing.

- Book a massage.

7-DAY RESTORE MENU

Prepare ahead

Vegetable stock (page 192)
Roast chicken (pages 187–8)
Chicken stock (pages 187–8)
Bone broth/Seaweed broth (V) (pages 191/189)
Nourish bites (page 173)
White kimchi (page 184)
Overnight oats (page 166)

Day 1

Lemon juice and hot water
Bircher overnight oats (pages 166–7)
Berry kefir booster (page 170)
Celeriac and umami mustard (2 batches) (page 130)
Nourish bite (page 173)
Sesame chicken/Corn, kale and avocado (V) (pages 156/89)

Day 2

Lemon juice and hot water
Almond chia smoothie (page 171)
Celeriac and umami mustard (page 130)
Chicken congee/Corn, kale and avocado (V) (pages 131/89)

Day 3

Lemon juice and hot water
Miso breakfast broth (page 169)
Nourish bite (optional) (page 173)
Ginger carrot with spiced coconut yoghurt (page 135)
Bone broth/Seaweed broth (V) (pages 191/189)
Magic soup (with optional kefir) (2 batches) (page 138)

Day 4

Lemon juice and hot water
Egg drop with nori (page 168)
Nourish bite (optional) (page 173)
Cumin-roasted sweet potato with onion and pomegranate molasses
(2 batches) (page 134)
Bone broth/Seaweed broth (V) (pages 191/189)
Magic soup (page 138)

Day 5

Lemon juice and hot water
Overnight oats with nuts and berries (pages 166-7)
Almond butter and apple on rye or nourish bite (page 173)
Cumin-roasted sweet potato with onion and pomegranate molasses
(page 134)
White kimchi (page 184)

Day 6

Lemon juice and hot water
Miso breakfast broth (page 169)
Sprouted soup (2 batches) (page 140)
Nourish bite (page 173)
Curried parsnip and apple (page 93)

Day 7

Lemon juice and hot water
Egg drop with nori (page 168)
Nourish bite (optional) (page 173)
Sprouted soup (page 140)
Bone broth/Seaweed broth (V) (pages 191/189)
Cod laksa/Curried parsnip and apple (V) (pages 133/93)

RENEW

5-DAY ENERGISING CLEANSE

GOALS

- Replenish energy reserves
- Wake up with vitality
- Grab life with both hands

This cleanse is like a tonic. Whether you are beginning to feel stressed out, finding it hard to jump out of bed in the morning or have that feeling of being tired most of the time, a cleanse is a helpful way to replenish your reserves and renew your sense of vitality. In this cleanse we have included a balance of calming foods with foods that in Chinese medicine are described as 'essence' foods.

Stress is one of the biggest challenges when it comes to sticking with our healthy intentions. Kate remembers working on a book all about healthy eating and finding the deadlines so stress-inducing that her own diet and lifestyle went haywire. Stress is both physically and emotionally exhausting, so the last thing we want to do when we get home is to cook from scratch. It's all to easy to just pour a glass of wine, flop on the couch and order a takeaway or eat a bag of crisps. For this cleanse, therefore, it is a great idea to clear the weekend of any commitments so that you can prepare some recipes for the week ahead.

Notes for the RENEW cleanse:

- Avoid processed or refined sugar.

- Avoid stimulants.

- Relax in the evenings and get to bed nice and early.

- As soon as you wake in the morning, get up.

- Meditation is great for this cleanse.

- Try energising movement exercise such as qi gong or lots of gentle walking to get your 'qi' moving.

5-DAY RENEW MENU

Prepare ahead

Roast chicken (pages 187–8)
Chicken stock (pages 187–8)
Vegetable stock (page 192)
Seaweed broth (page 189)/Bone broth (page 191)
Bircher museli (2 batches) (page 167)
Turmeric and black pepper oatcakes (page 175)

Day 1

Lemon juice and hot water
Dandelion tea
Bircher museli (page 167)
Sesame chicken/Sprouted soup (V) (pages 156/140)
Asparagus mimosa with two turmeric and black pepper oatcakes
(pages 104/175)

Day 2

Lemon juice and hot water
Dandelion tea
Bircher museli (page 167)
Chicken and nettle tops or Coconut chicken with turmeric and kale/
Sprouted soup (V) (page 147 or 106/140)
Squash and almond butter (2 batches) (page 158)

Day 3

Lemon juice and hot water
Nettle tea
Egg drop with nori (page 168)
Squash and almond butter (page 158)
Bone broth/Seaweed broth (V) (pages 191/189)
Beetroot and caraway (2 batches) with two turmeric and black
pepper oatcakes (pages 145/175)

Day 4

Lemon juice and hot water
Nettle tea
Berry kefir booster (page 170)
Beetroot and caraway with kale crisps (pages 145/174)
Bone broth/Seaweed broth (V) (pages 191/189)
Harissa broth with aubergine and quinoa (2 batches) (page 149)

Day 5

Lemon juice and hot water
Dandelion tea
Avocado on rye or gluten-free toast
Harissa broth with aubergine and quinoa (page 149)
Fennel-crusted salmon with ginger Chinese cabbage/Sopa de quinoa (V) (pages 148/157)

CHAPTER 6:
THE SOUPS

All calorie counts are per single serving.

RESOLVE

AVOCADO, LEMON, TURMERIC AND CAYENNE

Avocados are high in heart-healthy monounsaturated fatty acids (MUFAs) and fibre, making us feel fuller for longer. Peeling avocados means you get more of the nutrients close to the skin.

SERVES 1

163 kcal

¹/₂ ripe Hass avocado, peeled and stoned
100ml coconut milk
pinch of sea salt flakes
pinch of cayenne pepper
¹/₄ tsp ground turmeric
pinch of freshly ground black pepper
zest and juice of ¹/₂ small lemon (¹/₄ large)

Scoop out the flesh of the avocado into a blender with half the coconut milk and process until smooth. Add the rest of the coconut milk in stages until you reach your preferred consistency.

Add the salt, cayenne pepper, turmeric, black pepper, lemon zest and juice and blend again. Taste to check the flavour, and if you are happy with it, pour the soup into a container. Squeeze a bit more lemon juice over and cover the top of the soup with parchment, pressing it down to try to exclude air (to reduce discolouration).

Chill in the refrigerator before serving. If you want to serve immediately, add a couple of ice cubes when blending to chill the soup.

CORN, KALE AND AVOCADO

The coconut and chilli give the perfect punch to this combo. As part of the cruciferous family, kale is a rich source of antioxidants and has anti-inflammatory properties. Steaming kale is thought to maximise its nutritional benefits.

SERVES 2

1 corn on the cob (or
   use 100g frozen
   sweetcorn)
1 tbsp coconut oil
$\frac{1}{2}$ tsp chilli flakes
100g kale, thick stalks
   removed, leaves
   shredded
400ml hot vegetable or
   chicken stock (pages
   192 or 187–8
1 medium Hass avocado,
   peeled, stoned and
   sliced, to serve

Boil the corn on the cob in a pan of boiling unsalted water (salt will toughen the kernels) for 3–6 minutes or until cooked. Drain and allow to cool, then remove the kernels with a sharp knife.

Steam the kale for about 5 minutes.

Heat the coconut oil in a heavy-based pan and sauté the corn kernels with the chilli flakes for a couple of minutes before adding the kale and continuing to sauté for another 3–4 minutes. Add the hot stock and bring to the boil, then reduce to a simmer for a minute to bring the flavours together. Taste for seasoning.

Ladle the soup into bowls and top with sliced avocado.

BALTI-SPICED CAULIFLOWER

'Balti' spice is simply a mix of spices used in Indian cooking. Spices can be great for nourishing the digestive system, so adding them to your cooking is an easy way to improve your diet.

SERVES 2

FOR THE BALTI SPICE

1 tsp cumin seeds
1 tsp coriander seeds
$1/_2$ tsp fenugreek seeds
$1/_4$ tsp chilli flakes
$1/_2$ tsp ground turmeric
1 tsp paprika

FOR THE SOUP

2 tbsp olive oil
1 tsp balti spice
1 small or $1/_2$ large
    cauliflower (approx
    500g), cut into very
    small florets
200ml hot vegetable or
    chicken stock (pages
    192 or 187–8)
Saffron yoghurt (page
    185), to serve
    (optional)

First make the balti spice. Dry fry the cumin, coriander and fenugreek seeds for a couple of minutes and then grind with the chilli flakes in a spice grinder or pestle and mortar. Mix with the ground turmeric and paprika. Transfer to an airtight jar as you can keep the spice mix for months to use with other soups and vegetables.

To make the soup, heat the olive oil in a heavy-based pan and add 1 teaspoon of the spice mix. As the aromas are released, after about 30 seconds, add the cauliflower florets and stir through the spiced oil. Sauté the cauliflower for a couple of minutes before adding the hot stock. Bring to the boil and then reduce the heat. Check the cauliflower is cooked but still has a little bite. Switch off the heat.

To serve, ladle the soup into bowls and top with a spoonful of saffron yoghurt, if using.

BEETROOT, COCONUT AND SALMON

Herbalists call beetroot the 'vitality plant' – it is intensely nourishing and contains antioxidants, magnesium and iron, hardly any fat, very few calories and lots of fibre. The salmon is a great source of healthy omega-3 essential fatty acids and plenty of protein, so a bowl of this soup is packed with good nutrition.

SERVES 2

307 kcal

2 tsp coconut oil, plus extra (optional)
1 red onion, peeled and diced
1–2cm piece of fresh root ginger, peeled and finely chopped
1 garlic clove, peeled and finely chopped
250g beetroot, peeled and roughly chopped
200ml hot vegetable stock (page 192)
1 salmon fillet (skin on)
400ml canned light coconut milk

Heat the coconut oil in a heavy-based pan and add the onion. Sauté until soft, adding the ginger and garlic after 5 minutes. Add the beetroot to the pan and continue to cook for another 5 minutes, before adding the hot vegetable stock. Bring to the boil and then reduce to a simmer for about 30 minutes, or until the beetroot is cooked.

Meanwhile, steam or poach the salmon until it flakes easily. If you like, remove the skin, cut it into long strips and fry it in coconut oil over a high heat until crispy.

Add the coconut milk to the soup and simmer for a further 5 minutes. Whiz with a hand-held blender or in a food processor until smooth.

Serve in bowls with a handful of the flaked salmon and few strips of skin, for crunch, in the middle of the bowl.

CHICKEN SOUP FOR THE CLEANSED SOUL

The combination of slow-cooked chicken and spices (which aid your digestion) with the fresh peas, crunchy beansprouts and Chinese leaf (an antioxidant and anti-inflammatory) work so well together.

SERVES 2

1/2 tsp ground turmeric
1 tsp fennel seeds
pinch of chilli flakes
1 tbsp groundnut oil
2 large chicken thighs
hot chicken stock
    (pages 187–8)
    enough to cover the
    chicken pieces
2 garlic cloves, bashed
a few curry leaves
a couple of bay leaves
a few strands of
    lemon peel
50g fresh peas
50g beansprouts
50g Chinese leaf,
    shredded

Combine the turmeric, fennel seeds, chilli flakes and groundnut oil in a large mixing bowl and toss the chicken pieces in the spice mix.

Seal the chicken thighs in a hot saucepan, then add the hot chicken stock, bashed garlic, curry leaves, bay leaves and lemon peel. Simmer gently, uncovered, until the meat easily comes off the bone, about 45 minutes to 1 hour.

Remove the chicken from the stock and remove the meat. Return the shredded chicken to the stock along with the fresh peas, beansprouts and Chinese leaf and heat through. Divide the soup between two bowls.

CURRIED PARSNIP AND APPLE

This is naturally sweet and comforting for the colder months, while coconut milk is the perfect alternative to cream. Root vegetables are a rich source of fibre and easy on the digestion. It's good to remember that they draw their nutrients from the earth, reminding us of the importance of taking care of the soil.

SERVES 2

1 tbsp olive oil
1 large parsnip (scrubbed
    if organic, peeled if
    not), chopped
1 tsp garam masala
200ml hot vegetable
    stock (page 192)
100ml coconut milk
1 apple, cored and sliced,
    to serve
1 tbsp coconut oil
sea salt flakes and
    freshly ground black
    pepper, to taste

Heat the oil in a heavy-based pan and add the parsnip. Sauté for a couple of minutes, then create a space on the bottom of the pan and add the garam masala. Cook for about 30 seconds, until the aromas are released from the spices, then stir through the parsnip. Add the vegetable stock and some boiling water, if needed, to cover the parsnip. Bring to the boil, then reduce the heat and simmer for about 15 minutes. Add the coconut milk, then bring back to a simmer and cook until the parsnip is soft, about 30 minutes.

Allow the soup to cool a little, then whiz with a hand-held blender or in a food processor until smooth. Check for seasoning.

For the garnish, simply sauté the apple slices in a pan with the coconut oil until golden, then serve on top of the soup.

GREEN GAZPACHO

This chilled green soup is very cooling, so it's perfect for a hot summer's day.

SERVES 2

50g baby spinach

1/2 cucumber, peeled,
   deseeded and
   chopped

small handful of
   fresh basil

small handful of
   fresh mint

1/2 avocado, peeled
   and stoned

pinch of cayenne pepper

100g natural yoghurt
   or kefir

1 tbsp apple
   cider vinegar

1 tbsp extra virgin
   olive oil

2 breakfast radishes,
   thinly sliced, and
   radish sprouts,
   to serve

sea salt and freshly
   ground black pepper,
   to taste

Put all the ingredients, except the radishes, into a food processor and blend until smooth – you may need to add a little water to create your preferred consistency. Taste for seasoning.

To serve, divide among bowls and scatter over the radish slices and sprouts.

HOT CUCUMBER WITH SALMON

Salmon and cucumber is a classic combination, and cucumber is one of the best cleanse ingredients as it is a mild diuretic and helps the body get rid of excess water. It is naturally hydrating and the skin is full of fibre.

SERVES 2

300ml chicken stock
(pages 187–8)
300ml vegetable stock
(page 192)
1 lemongrass stalk,
bashed
1 skinless salmon fillet
1 small cucumber,
deseeded and sliced
3 spring onions, chopped
1 tbsp tamari wheat-free
soy sauce
fresh root ginger, peeled
and thinly sliced,
to serve

Bring all the stock to the boil in a pan then reduce the heat to a good simmer. Add the lemongrass and simmer for 10 minutes. Steam the salmon fillet in a steamer set on top of the stock pan for 3 minutes, then take it off the heat. Keep the salmon in the covered steamer for another 5 minutes.

Remove the lemongrass from the stock using a slotted spoon, then add the cucumber, spring onions and tamari. Flake the salmon into bowls, pour over the aromatic soup, and serve with fresh ginger slices scattered over.

HOT CUCUMBER
WITH BARLEY

In this vegetarian version of the previous soup, the barley takes central stage. This grain is a good home remedy for water retention so this soup is perfect for when you feel bloated.

SERVES 2

600ml vegetable stock
(page 192)
1 lemongrass stalk,
bashed
80g pearl barley
1 small cucumber,
deseeded and sliced
3 spring onions, chopped
1 green chilli, thinly
sliced
1 tbsp tamari wheat-free
soy sauce
fresh root ginger,
peeled and thinly
sliced, to serve

Bring the stock to the boil in a pan and reduce the heat to a good simmer. Add the lemongrass and pearl barley. Cover, leaving a bit of a gap between the lid and pan so the stock doesn't boil over. Once the barley is tender, about 45 minutes, take the pan off the heat and remove the lemongrass.

Stir in the cucumber, spring onions, chilli and tamari. Serve with fresh ginger slices scattered over.

LEEK, FENNEL AND CELERY WITH RED LENTILS

The vegetables in this soup have diuretic properties so help resolve excess water in the body or 'damp' as Chinese medicine aptly describes it.

SERVES 2

237 kcal

1 leek

1 celery heart (keep
    outer part for stock)

inner leaves of 1 fennel
    (keep outer part
    for stock)

1 tbsp olive oil

200ml hot vegetable
    stock (page 192)

200g dried red lentils,
    thoroughly rinsed

½ preserved lemon,
    finely chopped

Chop the leek, celery and fennel into equally sized small cubes – a mirepoix. Heat the olive oil in a heavy-based pan and sauté the vegetables for about 10 minutes, until soft.

Add the hot vegetable stock and lentils, bring to the boil, then reduce the heat to a simmer for about 20 minutes. Add the preserved lemon, stir through and then take the soup off the heat. Ideally, allow the soup to sit overnight as it improves as the flavours infuse.

To serve, warm through and enjoy.

SPICED COD WITH SAMPHIRE

You can use any white fish for this recipe. Seashore nutrition is returning to our cooking and we have used samphire here, which grows on marshes close to the sea and contains phytochemicals that are protective of the liver.

SERVES 2

1 tbsp coconut oil

2.5cm piece of
   cinnamon stick

4 cloves

$1/2$ tsp mustard seeds

8 curry leaves

$1/2$ onion, peeled and
   thinly sliced

2 garlic cloves, crushed

1 tsp freshly
   grated ginger

$1/2$ tsp ground turmeric
   (or $1/4$ tsp grated
   turmeric root)

100ml vegetable stock
   (page 192)

100ml coconut milk

80g samphire, rinsed

200g cod fillets (or any
   firm white fish)

$1/2$ tsp white miso paste

squeeze of lime juice,
   to serve

Heat half the coconut oil in a heavy-based pan and fry the cinnamon, cloves, mustard seeds and curry leaves. When the aromas are released and the mustard seeds are just starting to pop, add the onion and sauté for 8–10 minutes before adding the crushed garlic, ginger and turmeric.

Meanwhile, bring the stock and coconut milk to the boil in a separate pan, then reduce the heat to a simmer. Pour the hot stock and coconut milk into the pan with the onions.

Heat the remaining coconut oil in a frying pan and sauté the samphire for a few minutes, then remove from the pan. Brush the fish fillets with white miso and fry, skin-side down, in the frying pan for about 5 minutes until almost cooked through. Turn over, and take off the heat. The fish will finish cooking in the residual heat.

To serve, ladle the coconut broth into bowls, flake over the fish and scatter over the samphire. Squeeze with the lime juice to serve.

SALMON POACHED IN LEMONGRASS TEA

This soup has plenty of clean flavours: the lemongrass, celery and raw vitality of the peppery radishes will all maximise your cleanse.

SERVES 2

large pot of hot
 lemongrass tea (about
 1 litre)
1 salmon fillet (about
 150g)
1 celery stalk, sliced
 lengthways into batons
small handful of
 radishes, thinly sliced
furikake seasoning
 or black and white
 sesame seeds
 (optional)
sea salt flakes and
 freshly ground black
 pepper, to taste

Bring half the tea up to the boil in a pan and add the salmon fillet. Reduce to a simmer and poach for about 8 minutes, or until the flesh is just nicely flaking. Remove the salmon and flake the flesh, discarding the skin.

Divide the celery and radishes between two serving bowls, add the salmon flakes, then pour over the remaining hot tea. Season with furikake or sesame seeds (if using), and salt and pepper, then serve.

SUMMER CHICKEN

This is a delicious way to enjoy fresh summer vegetables, with all the flavours brought together in a warming little broth.

SERVES 2

400ml chicken stock
(pages 187–8)
200g leftover roast
chicken, shredded
small handful of mint
leaves, shredded
50g broad beans, double
podded
50g fresh garden peas
2 small little gem lettuce,
shredded
2 tbsp natural yoghurt,
to serve

Bring the chicken stock to the boil in a pan, then reduce the heat to a simmer. Add the chicken pieces, mint, broad beans and garden peas – the soup will be ready to serve in just a minute. Taste for seasoning, ladle into bowls, and top with the little gem and natural yoghurt.

WILD GARLIC, BABY SPINACH AND OLIVE

Wild garlic, with its many sulphur compounds, helps to clear the inside of the digestive tract. It detoxifies the gut from pathogens and at the same time supports the 'good' bacteria. It kills many parasites and may assist in clearing Candida albicans, a common yeast infection. Wild garlic is a truly versatile and health-boosting plant.

SERVES 2

80g brown rice
1 tbsp olive oil
2 shallots, finely sliced
50g wild garlic, roughly
  chopped
50g baby spinach
50g Kalamata olives,
  stoned and sliced
500ml chicken or
  vegetable stock (pages
  187–8 or 192)

Cook the brown rice according to the packet instructions, then drain.

Meanwhile, heat the oil in a large frying pan or wok, add the shallots and sauté for a few minutes until soft. Add in the wild garlic and cook for a couple of minutes before adding the baby spinach and olives. Give everything a good stir and cook until the spinach is just wilted.

Meanwhile, heat the stock in a large pan. Divide the cooked rice between two bowls and top with the wild garlic, spinach and olives, then ladle over the hot stock.

REBALANCE

ASPARAGUS MIMOSA

This soup is very seasonal, perfect for late spring. Asparagus contains a number of anti-inflammatory nutrients, and like Jerusalem artichoke has prebiotic properties, making it supportive to digestive health.

SERVES 2

241 kcal

1 egg
¼ celery stalk, finely
    chopped
250g white or green
    asparagus spears
1 tbsp olive oil
500ml hot vegetable or
    chicken stock
    (pages 192 or 187–8)
2 tbsp natural yoghurt
sea salt, to taste

Boil the egg in a pan of boiling water for 8 minutes (from the water boiling), then cool under running water, peel and chop. Mix the egg with the chopped celery, then season with a pinch of sea salt.

To make the soup, snap off the woody parts of the asparagus (keep them for making stock) and chop the spears into 2.5cm pieces. Heat the oil in a pan, add the asparagus and sauté for 2 minutes before adding enough stock to cover. Bring to the boil, then reduce the heat to a simmer and cook until the asparagus pieces are tender, which should only take a few minutes. Blend the asparagus with enough stock to make a smooth soup and check the seasoning.

Stir the yoghurt through the soup and divide it between two bowls. Serve with the chopped egg and celery scattered over the top.

CHICKEN AND COURGETTE THAI NOODLE SOUP

Courgettes are so plentiful in late summer and are a good source of antioxidants in the form of carotenoids. Simply use a potato peeler to cut the courgette into ribbons.

SERVES 2

1 tbsp coconut oil
1 tbsp Thai paste
(page 181)
1 large or 2 small
carrots, grated
150ml chicken stock
(pages 187–8)
200ml canned coconut
milk (¹/₂ x 400ml can)
200g leftover roast
chicken, shredded
1 courgette, cut into
ribbons
small handful of Thai
basil leaves, to serve

Heat the coconut oil in a large saucepan or wok, add the Thai paste and, a few seconds later, add the grated carrot and stir through. After a minute or so, add the stock and coconut milk, bring to the boil, then reduce the heat to a simmer.

Add the chicken pieces and courgette to the pan and warm through. Take off the heat and let the flavours infuse for a couple of minutes before serving in deep bowls, scattered with Thai basil leaves.

COCONUT CHICKEN WITH TURMERIC AND KALE

Turmeric, kale and coconut oil happen to work beautifully together and this hearty soup is packed with cleansing benefits.

SERVES 1

378 kcal

½ onion, chopped
1 tbsp coconut oil, melted
150ml coconut water
100ml chicken stock (pages 187–8)
1 tsp ground turmeric or ¼ tsp fresh turmeric, grated
50g kale, tough stalks removed and leaves shredded
½ tbsp pumpkin seeds
80g leftover roast chicken, shredded
squeeze of lemon juice, to taste (optional)
freshly ground black pepper, to taste

In a heavy-based pan, sauté the onion in half the coconut oil until soft. Add the coconut water, turmeric and some freshly ground black pepper.

Heat the remaining oil in a frying pan or wok and sauté the kale for a few minutes until softened slightly, then add the pumpkin seeds and stir through.

Place the kale and shredded chicken in a bowl and pour over the hot coconut water. Taste it – it might need a squeeze of lemon.

COURGETTE, LEMON AND THYME

In our cookbook, Magic Soup, we included a courgette and za'atar soup, which is both delicious and very quick and easy to prepare. Za'atar isn't always easy to find; it's a Middle Eastern blend made from the herb za'atar that is grown in Lebanon – which is similar to thyme in flavour – and blended with sumac and sesame seeds. Here is our simplified version of that recipe using easy-to-find ingredients.

SERVES 2

188 kcal

2 tbsp light olive oil
300g courgettes (about 3–4), cut into cubes
1 tsp fresh thyme leaves, picked and finely chopped
zest of $\frac{1}{2}$ lemon
300ml hot chicken or vegetable stock (pages 187–8 or 192)
1 tbsp pumpkin seeds

Heat the oil in a heavy-based pan and cook the courgettes gently for about 3 minutes. Stir in the thyme and half the lemon zest.

Add the hot stock, bring to a boil, then reduce the heat to a simmer and cook gently until the courgettes are cooked but not too soft.

In the meantime, heat a non-stick frying pan and dry fry the pumpkin seeds with the remainder of the lemon zest until they just begin to pop a little – keep shaking the pan to prevent them burning.

Remove the courgettes from the heat and allow to cool a little before blending half of them in a food processor with as much stock from the pan as you need to reach the desired consistency (you may prefer a smooth or slightly textured soup).

Divide the remaining courgettes between two bowls, creating a pyramid in the middle. Ladle the blended soup around the courgettes and sprinkle with the toasted pumpkin seeds.

FIVE-SPICE TOFU

Organic tofu is an excellent source of vegetarian protein and takes on any spice or herb flavours that you fancy. Buckwheat or brown rice noodles are a lovely addition to this soup.

SERVES 2

146 kcal

200g firm fresh tofu, drained and cut into 2cm cubes

¹/₂ tsp mustard seeds, crushed

¹/₂ tsp black onion seeds, crushed

¹/₄ tsp sea salt flakes

¹/₂ tsp Chinese five-spice powder

1 tsp white miso paste

1 tbsp coconut oil, melted

100g mixed leafy greens, such as bok choy, Swiss chard, kale, tatsoi or cabbage, finely sliced

Put the tofu cubes in a large mixing bowl with the crushed mustard seeds, black onion seeds, salt flakes and five-spice and toss to coat.

Dissolve the white miso paste in 400ml just-boiled water from the kettle.

Heat the coconut oil in a frying pan, add the greens and sauté gently for 2–3 minutes, until tender. Layer the greens and tofu in serving bowls or large glass Kilner jars, pour over the white miso broth, then serve.

HARISSA CAULIFLOWER AND CORN

Cauliflower is a blank canvas for taking on flavour. It's the perfect ingredient for soup that satisfies.

SERVES 2

239 kcal

1 tbsp olive oil
$\frac{1}{2}$ medium onion, peeled and finely chopped
1 tsp rose harissa paste
$\frac{1}{2}$ medium cauliflower (about 500g), cut into small florets
300ml hot vegetable stock (page 192)
1 corn on the cob, steamed or boiled, kernels removed (or use frozen)

Heat the oil in a heavy-based pan and sauté the onion until soft and translucent, about 10 minutes. Add the rose harissa and stir into the onion, then add the cauliflower florets and stir through.

After a couple of minutes, add the hot vegetable stock and simmer for 7–10 minutes, or until the cauliflower is cooked but still has a little bite. Add the cooked corn kernels and heat through.

Process half the soup in a blender, then check for seasoning. Divide the blended soup between two bowls and top with the remaining unblended soup.

HORSERADISH AND LEMONY SQUASH

The mustardy spice of the horseradish, used as a herbal remedy for colds, is perfect with the sweetness of the butternut squash.

SERVES 2

2 tbsp olive oil
500g butternut squash,
    peeled, deseeded
    and cut into small
    equal cubes
¹/₂ tsp fresh horseradish,
    grated (or 1 tsp from
    a jar)
zest of ¹/₂ lemon
300ml hot chicken or
    vegetable stock
    (pages 187–8 and 192)
50ml almond milk
small handful of fresh
    tarragon
1 tbsp cleanse dukkah
    (page 183)

Heat the olive oil in a heavy-based pan and sauté the squash for about 5 minutes. Stir through the horseradish and lemon zest, before adding the hot stock. Bring to the boil, then reduce the heat to a simmer until the squash is cooked, 5–10 minutes.

Take off the heat and remove some of the squash cubes with a slotted spoon. Set aside. Add the almond milk and tarragon to the squash-and-stock mix and blend in a food processor until smooth.

To serve, divide the soup between two bowls and spoon in the diced squash. Scatter over the cleanse dukkah.

KITCHARI

This recipe for kitchari is based on the ancient medicine tradition of Ayurveda. This is a soup that will get rid of any bloating or water retention and have you feeling light on your toes in no time.

SERVES 2

219 kcal

100g green mung beans
1 tsp ground turmeric
$^1/_4$ tsp asafoetida
2 tbsp coconut oil, melted
1 tsp cleanse spice mix (page 183)
zest and juice of 1 lime
sea salt flakes and freshly ground black pepper, to taste
Greek yoghurt, to serve

Rinse the mung beans in several changes of water, then leave to soak in a bowl of water overnight. Rinse and drain the beans again and put them in a saucepan with 1 litre of fresh water. Bring to the boil, add the turmeric and asafoetida, then reduce the heat to a simmer and cook gently for 45 minutes to 1 hour, until the beans are soft.

Heat half the coconut oil in a frying pan and add the cleanse spices and lime zest. Fry until the aromas are released, then add to the soup along with the lime juice. Check for seasoning, add the remaining coconut oil and put the lid on. Take off the heat and let the soup stand for 10 minutes.

Serve with a spoonful of yoghurt.

LEMON, CHICKEN AND MINT

Lemon juice is thought to be beneficial for the digestion, which is why it's a good start to the day. The pectin found in lemon peel is a particularly good source of fibre that helps you to feel satisfied after a meal.

SERVES 2

174 kcal

800ml chicken stock
(pages 187–8)
2 boneless, skinless
chicken thighs (or
150g leftover cooked
chicken, shredded)
zest and juice of
1 unwaxed lemon,
zest cut into thin strips
handful of fresh mint
leaves, chopped

Bring the chicken stock to the boil in a large pan, then add the chicken thighs, lemon zest and mint (reserve about 1 tablespoon of mint for serving). Poach gently for 10–15 minutes or until the chicken is cooked through. Remove the chicken from the pan, leave it to cool a little, then slice or pull it into thin strips. (If you are using leftover cooked chicken, simmer just the lemon peel and mint in the stock to infuse the flavours.)

Bring the broth back to a simmer and return the chicken to the pan along with the juice of half the lemon. Taste to see if you need more.

To serve, stir through the reserved chopped mint and ladle the soup into bowls.

PEA AND PRESERVED LEMON

*As part of the legumes family (foods that come from a pod), green peas
are a great source of antioxidants and are convenient to have on hand for a
five-minute soup. This is also delicious with cottage cheese when you aren't
on a cleanse.*

SERVES 1

134
kcal

100ml chicken stock
(pages 187–8)
pinch of chilli flakes
100g frozen peas
30g Greek yoghurt, plus
extra to serve
1 tsp preserved lemon,
finely chopped
handful of fresh dill,
chopped

Boil the chicken stock with the chilli flakes in
a pan then reduce to a simmer. Add the peas
and simmer for a couple of minutes or until
they are cooked but still have a little bite.

Mix the Greek yoghurt, preserved lemon and
dill together. To serve, either leave the peas
whole or blend to a smooth soup with a
hand-held blender or in a food processor
and ladle into bowls. Add a few small
spoonfuls of the yoghurt on top to serve.

ROASTED CHERRY TOMATO AND LEMON SOUP WITH SALSA

Tomatoes are one of the best sources of heart-and-bone-healthy lycopene. They are also a taste of summer.

SERVES 2 *133 kcal*

500g mixed heritage or cherry tomatoes, on the vine
1 tbsp olive oil
1 tbsp balsamic vinegar
1 tsp grated unwaxed lemon zest
$\frac{1}{2}$ tbsp capers, rinsed, drained and chopped
1 spring onion, thinly sliced
200ml hot vegetable stock (page 192)
1 tbsp tomato purée
sea salt flakes, to taste
flatbreads, to serve (optional)

Preheat the oven to 230°C/450°F/gas mark 8.

Arrange 400g of the tomatoes in a single layer on a baking tray, leaving them on the vine. Drizzle with the olive oil and balsamic vinegar, sprinkle with the lemon zest and season with a little sea salt. Roast for about 10 minutes, until the tomatoes are bursting. Now switch off the oven and allow the tomatoes to continue to soften in the residual heat.

Meanwhile, make the salsa by chopping the remaining cherry tomatoes and mixing them with the capers and spring onion.

Remove the roasted cherry tomatoes from the vines, put them in a blender or a food processor with the hot stock and tomato purée and blend until smooth.

To serve, either garnish the soup with the salsa or serve it on the side with wheat-free seeded flatbreads. We have fallen in love with chickpea flatbreads: perfect for the salsa. We have fallen in love with chickpea flatbreads: perfect for the salsa.

SAFFRON BROTH WITH FISH

Saffron is mostly associated with risotto but when you simply allow it to infuse in a broth its flavour really shines.

SERVES 2

133 kcal

75g baby leeks
75g baby carrots
75g baby fennel
500ml vegetable stock
   (page 192)
a few strands of saffron
200g white fish or
   cooked prawns
sea salt flakes and
   freshly ground black
   pepper, to taste
squeeze of lemon,
   to serve

Top and tail the baby vegetables and add to a pan along with the vegetable stock, the saffron and a good pinch of sea salt. Bring to the boil, reduce the heat and simmer until the vegetables are cooked and still have a nice bite. Taste for seasoning.

To cook the fish, simply steam until flaky.

To serve, ladle the broth into bowls and flake in the fish or scatter over the prawns, or simply enjoy the vegetables and broth by themselves. Add a little more sea salt, freshly ground black pepper and a squeeze of lemon juice over the fish or prawns.

SICHUAN PEPPER AND CHICKEN

We have noticed many of the Western trends in healthy food have their roots in ancient Eastern traditions including Ayurveda and Chinese medicine. Sichuan peppers from China are said to warm the body, reduce 'damp', and support digestion.

SERVES 2

268 kcal

500ml seaweed broth (page 189)

6 spring onions, 3 cut into 2cm pieces, 3 finely sliced

1/2 thumb-sized piece fresh root ginger, peeled and thinly sliced

2 star anise

1/2 tbsp Sichuan peppercorns

1 tbsp tamari wheat-free soy sauce

2 large boneless, skinless, chicken thighs (or leftover roast chicken)

100g collard or turnip greens, rinsed, stems removed and shredded

1 tbsp light sesame oil

Bring the seaweed broth to the boil in a pan, then reduce the heat to a good simmer and add the spring onions, ginger, star anise, Sichuan peppercorns and tamari. Simmer for about 15 minutes to infuse the stock.

Add the chicken thighs (but not the cooked chicken if using leftovers) and poach for about 10 minutes, or until cooked through. Remove from the stock and allow to cool before pulling them apart into smaller pieces.

Sauté the collard greens in a frying pan with a little light sesame oil.

Pass the stock through a sieve into a clean pan and add the chicken pieces and greens. Taste for seasoning before ladling into individual bowls.

SMOKED AUBERGINE AND KEFIR

Inspired by working with Yotam Ottolenghi, Nicole was happy to discover that aubergine is surprisingly low in calories. It's a great vegetarian alternative to meat with its rich texture and taste. By cooking it on the flame you don't need to add any oil but you should discard the charred skin.

SERVES 2

2 aubergines
100ml kefir
100ml vegetable stock
    (page 192)
1 garlic clove
1 tbsp natural yoghurt
zest of $\frac{1}{2}$ lime
extra virgin olive oil and
    rye bread, to serve

To smoke your aubergines, simply cook them directly over the gas flame, holding them carefully with long-handled tongs and turning them as the skin chars on each side until the flesh is soft within. When they are completely charred and softened, place them in a bowl and cover until cool – this makes them very easy to peel. Once cooked, peel, remove the seeds and discard both the skin and seeds.

Bring the kefir, vegetable stock and garlic to the boil in a pan. Add the aubergine flesh, reduce the heat to a simmer and cook for 10 minutes. Allow to cool slightly before whizzing in a blender or food processor along with the yoghurt and lime zest.

Serve drizzled with extra virgin olive oil and with a slice of rye bread alongside.

HOT SMOKED MUSHROOM

Smoking the mushrooms is optional here. As a chef, Nicole would happily smoke anything; at home, we just use a large roasting tray that has a lid. You lay a mixture of tea leaves and rice on the bottom of the tray (Earl grey is great, or green), pop a rack over the top and put whatever you are smoking on the rack. Cover the tray with the lid and turn on the hob to a high heat. Set the tray over the heat and when it starts to smoke (check every minute or so by having a look under the lid), lower the heat. If you don't fancy smoking the mushrooms, you can sauté everything together, just adding a little more coconut oil.

SERVES 2

100g button mushrooms
1 tbsp coconut oil
100g chestnut
    mushrooms, sliced
1 garlic clove, crushed
50ml almond milk
100ml hot vegetable or
    chicken stock (pages
    192 or 187–8)

If you are smoking the mushrooms, load up your smoking tray or pan as described above and smoke the button mushrooms for about 35 minutes.

Heat the coconut oil in a pan and sauté the chestnut mushrooms until soft, adding the garlic after a minute or two. Deglaze the pan with the almond milk and then add the hot stock and simmer for a few minutes.

Add the smoked mushrooms to the pan before blending the soup in a blender or food processor to your desired consistency.

SPINACH AND SPICED ONION

*Adding quinoa to vegetables before blending not only creates a creamy
texture without the need for cream but also adds a good amount of protein.*

SERVES 2

1 tbsp coconut oil,
   melted
1 medium onion, peeled
   and sliced
1/4 tsp ground cloves
80g quinoa
400ml hot vegetable
   stock (page 192)
200g baby spinach
20g fresh basil leaves
sea salt and freshly
   ground black pepper,
   to taste
2 tbsp natural yoghurt,
   to serve (optional)

Heat the coconut oil in a heavy-based pan
and add the onion. Gently sauté for about
10 minutes until soft and starting to turn
golden. Make a space in the pan and add the
ground cloves. After a few seconds, as the
aroma of the cloves is released, stir through
the onions and continue to cook for a minute.
Leave half the onions in the pan and reserve
the rest.

Add the quinoa to the pan with the
vegetable stock. Simmer for about 15
minutes. Take off the heat before adding the
baby spinach and basil. Whiz the soup
in a blender or food processor until smooth
and check for seasoning. To serve, reheat the
reserved onions, ladle the soup into bowls
and top with the onions and yoghurt, if using.

SPRING CHICKEN

This is the perfect mid-week meal to use up your leftover roast chicken with some crunchy spring cabbage and spicy mustard.

SERVES 2

1 tbsp groundnut oil

$^1/_2$ spring cabbage, finely shredded

200g leftover roast chicken, shredded

1 tbsp umami mustard (page 182) or grain mustard

400ml hot chicken stock (pages 187–8)

sea salt and freshly ground black pepper, to taste

Heat the oil in a wok and when beginning to smoke add the cabbage and stir-fry for a couple of minutes. Add the chicken and stir through the mustard for another half minute before adding the hot stock. Bring to the boil, then reduce the heat to a gentle simmer and cook for a few minutes to let the flavours infuse. Check for seasoning and serve.

TOFU SEA SPAGHETTI MISO

This is a great store cupboard dish that you can add to, depending on what fresh ingredients you have to hand.

SERVES 1

340 kcal

100g fresh tofu, cubed
¹/₂ tsp ground turmeric
1 tbsp toasted sesame oil
20g sea spaghetti, rinsed
1 miso sachet

Marinate the tofu in the ground turmeric and sesame oil.

Bring a pan of water to the boil and add the sea spaghetti, reduce the heat to a simmer and cook for 5–10 minutes, or until the seaweed is al dente.

Make your miso soup according to the packet instructions and add the sea spaghetti and tofu. You may want to add some extra greens, such as baby spinach or baby kale, or a handful of beansprouts.

SMOKED TOFU, TOMATO AND BROCCOLI

Tofu adds a creaminess to the tomato soup base for this recipe, the perfect backdrop to the crunchy, deep green broccoli.

SERVES 2

100g large tomatoes, roughly chopped

100ml vegetable stock (page 192)

100g datterini (or cherry on the vine) tomatoes, chopped

50g sun-blushed tomatoes in olive oil, drained

50g smoked tofu

60g tenderstem broccoli

1 tsp hemp seeds

sea salt and freshly ground black pepper, to taste

Place the large tomatoes in a pan with the vegetable stock. Bring to the boil, then reduce to a simmer. Season with a little sea salt and freshly ground black pepper.

Add the datterini tomatoes and continue to simmer for 15 minutes. Finely chop half the sun-blushed tomatoes and add to the pan. Take off the heat and whiz with a blender or in a food processor with the tofu to a smooth soup, then pass it through a sieve.

Boil or steam the broccoli, drain, cool and then chop into bite-sized pieces. Place in a mixing bowl and add the remainder of the sun-blushed tomatoes, a drizzle of the tomato oil and the hemp seeds. Mix to combine.

Warm the soup, divide between bowls and top with the broccoli salad.

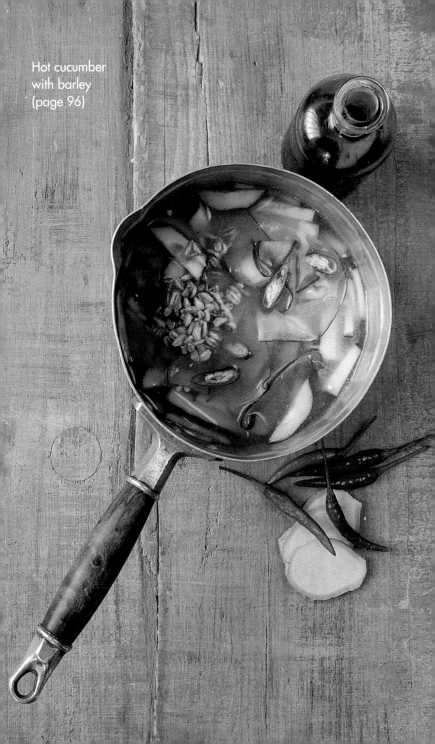

Hot cucumber
with barley
(page 96)

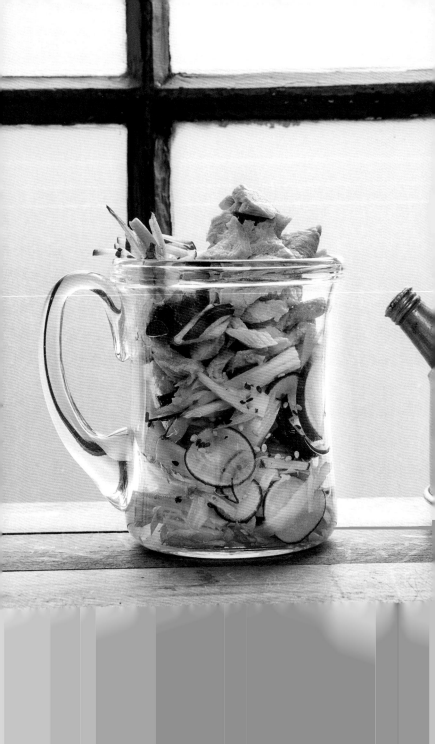

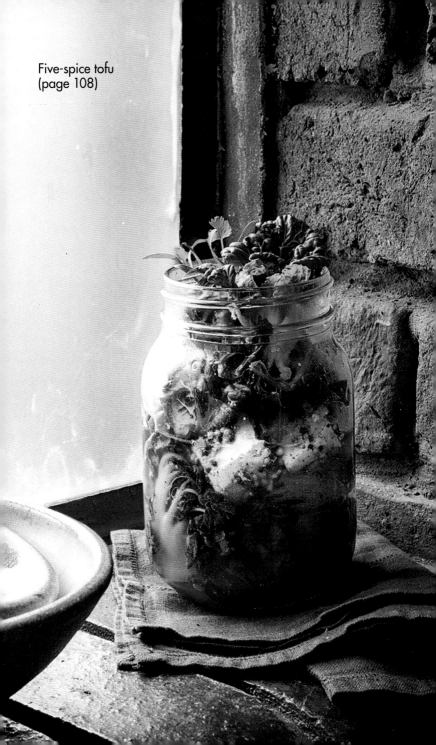

Five-spice tofu
(page 108)

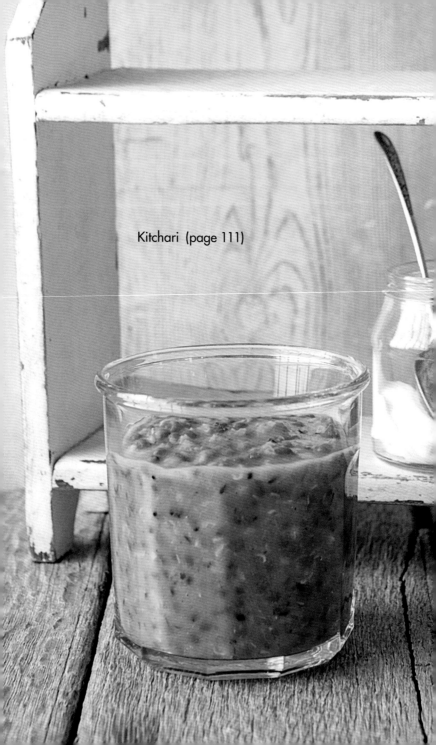

Kitchari (page 111)

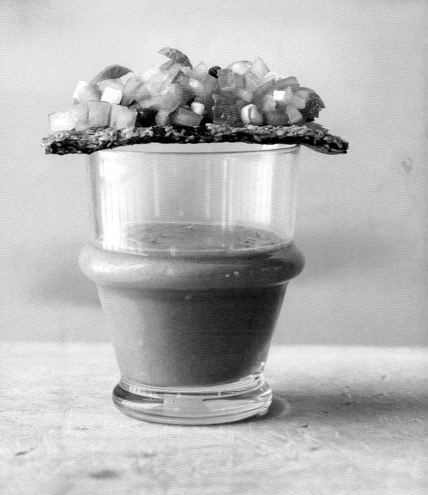

Roasted cherry tomato and lemon soup
with salsa (page 114)

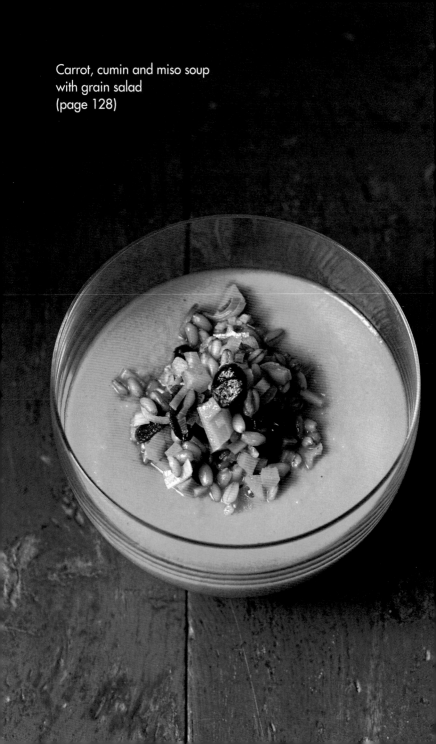

Carrot, cumin and miso soup
with grain salad
(page 128)

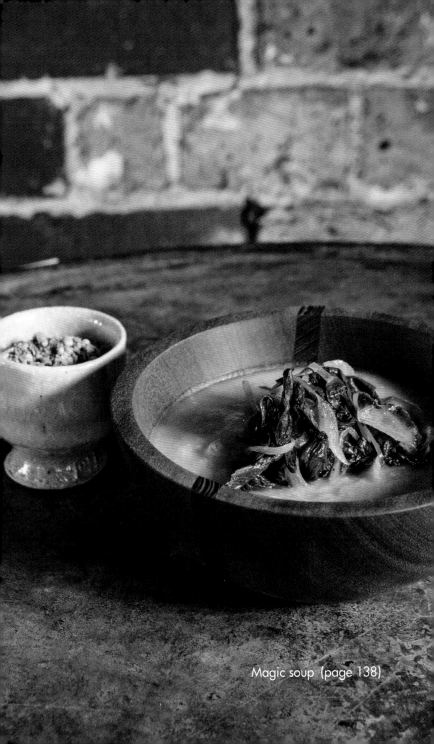

Magic soup (page 138)

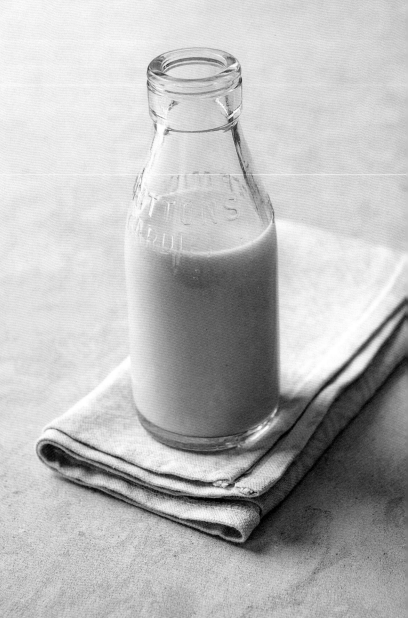

Raw soup (page 152)

RESTORE

AUTUMN CHICKEN

Mushrooms are a source of vitamin D and B vitamins, and studies suggest they may be beneficial for our immune system. They are a wonderful addition to autumn soups.

SERVES 2

266
kcal

1 tbsp groundnut oil
80g mushrooms
    (chanterelle,
    oyster, girolle)
400ml chicken stock
    (pages 187–8)
200g leftover roast
    chicken, shredded
small handful of
    tarragon, chopped
sea salt and freshly
    ground black pepper,
    to taste

Heat the oil in a frying pan and gently sauté the mushrooms until soft.

In a separate pan, heat the chicken stock and add the chicken pieces. Add the mushrooms to the soup and gently simmer for a couple of minutes. Check for seasoning and serve with chopped tarragon scattered over.

BUCKWHEAT BROTH

Buckwheat is a ancient plant that produces grain-like seeds that are an excellent gluten-free alternative to wheat. It contains protein and essential amino acids, and is also delicious in the form of soba noodles.

SERVES 2

600ml vegetable stock
(page 192)
1 lemongrass stalk,
bashed
100g buckwheat
100g kale, stalks
removed and
shredded
2cm piece of fresh root
ginger, peeled and
finely grated
pinch of chilli flakes
1 tbsp coconut oil,
melted
2 tbsp wheat-free tamari
soy sauce

In a pan, bring the vegetable stock to the boil and reduce to a simmer. Add the bashed lemongrass and the buckwheat. Once the buckwheat is tender (check the packet instructions for timings), take the pan off the heat and remove the lemongrass.

Sauté the shredded kale, ginger and chilli in a little coconut oil then add a good splash of tamari. To serve, divide the kale between bowls and ladle the buckwheat broth over.

BUTTERNUT SQUASH AND SAGE

Both butternet squash and sage are good for the digestion. Sage can also be used as a herbal remedy for sore throats and colds, so this soup is particularly useful for the cooler times of year.

SERVES 2 309 kcal

2 tbsp olive oil
6 large sage leaves
½ butternut squash, peeled, seeds removed and chopped
1 onion, peeled and quartered
400ml hot vegetable or chicken stock (pages 192 or 187–8)
sea salt and freshly ground black pepper, to taste
Greek yoghurt, to serve

Preheat the oven to 200°C/400°F/gas mark 6.

Heat the oil in a frying pan and add the sage leaves. When crispy, remove the leaves and dry on a piece of kitchen paper. Set aside for garnishing the soup later and keep the oil for the next step.

Place the squash pieces and onion in a large bowl and add the infused oil, combining thoroughly. Transfer to a roasting tray and roast in the oven for about 45 minutes until the squash is soft and slightly caramelised. Blend with the hot stock in batches until smooth. Taste for seasoning and serve with some Greek yoghurt and the crispy sage leaves.

CARDAMOM COCONUT BARLEY

This recipe is packed with digestion-friendly spices, lean protein and slow-release grains. It will keep you energised all day.

SERVES 2
386 kcal

50g coconut oil
50g grated fresh ginger
3 garlic cloves, crushed
10 curry leaves
1 green chilli, finely
  chopped
$1/4$ tsp finely grated
  fresh turmeric (or 1 tsp
  ground turmeric)
1 tsp cumin seeds
1 tsp fennel seeds
$1^1/_2$ tsp black mustard
  seeds
450ml coconut milk
6 cardamom pods
1 tbsp groundnut oil
80g turkey mince
75g cooked pearl barley
bunch of fresh coriander,
  chopped, to serve
bunch of spring onions,
  chopped, to serve

Melt the coconut oil in a non-stick pan then fry the ginger, garlic, curry leaves and chilli until fragrant. Add the turmeric, cumin seeds, fennel and black mustard seeds and continue to fry until the spices release their aromas and the mustard seeds just begin to pop.

Take off the heat and allow the mixture to cool before blending to a paste in a food processor or pestle and mortar.

Bring the coconut milk to the boil, crush and split the cardamom pods and add to the coconut milk. Simmer for 10 minutes to infuse, strain through a sieve to remove the pods, then discard them.

Heat the groundnut oil in a heavy-based saucepan and gently fry the turkey mince until cooked through, adding a tablespoon of the spice paste after a couple of minutes.

Add the infused coconut milk and the cooked barley and gently simmer for 5 minutes before serving in bowls scattered with plenty of chopped coriander and spring onion.

CARROT, CUMIN AND MISO SOUP WITH GRAIN SALAD

To help calm the mind you need to calm and gently nourish the digestion, as the two are intrinsically linked – hence all those phrases like 'food for thought'. The digestion likes naturally sweet foods such as carrots and squash, and also gentle aromatic herbs and spices such as cinnamon, cumin and basil, so for mindful soup go with the simplest soup of all: carrot and cumin.

SERVES 2

FOR THE SOUP

1 tbsp coconut oil, melted
$1/_2$ onion, sliced
$1/_2$ tsp cumin seeds
500g carrots, roughly chopped
$1/_2$ tsp white miso paste

FOR THE SALAD

50g freekeh (or buckwheat for wheat-free alternative)
10g dried cranberries, soaked in a little warm water for 10 minutes then drained
$1/_4$ onion, finely chopped
$1/_4$ celery stick, finely chopped
$1/_4$ carrot, finely chopped

Heat the coconut oil in a large pan, add the onion and cook for 10 minutes until soft. Push the onion to one side to create space in the pan and add the cumin seeds. When the seeds start to release their aroma, add the carrots and give everything a good stir. Add the miso paste and stir it in through the vegetables, then add 400ml of just-boiled water from the kettle. Bring to the boil, then simmer for 10 minutes, or until the carrots can be easily pierced with a sharp knife. Process the soup in a blender or food processor until smooth.

To make the salad, put the grains in a pan, cover with water and bring to the boil. Simmer until the grains are cooked (check the packet for instructions). When the grains are cooked, drain and mix them in a large bowl with the drained cranberries, onion, celery and carrot.

Serve the soup topped with a couple of spoonfuls of the grain salad.

CARROT, GINGER AND TANGERINE

This soup packs a vitamin C punch, and the carrot and ginger are warming and good for the digestion.

SERVES 2

146 kcal

1 tbsp olive oil
1/2 onion, peeled and
   sliced
1 celery stalk, sliced
4 carrots, scrubbed (if
   organic, peeled if not)
   and chopped
1/2 tsp grated fresh
   ginger
zest and juice of
   1 tangerine, cut
   into thin strips
400ml hot vegetable
   stock (page 192)
cleanse dukkah, to serve
   (page 183)

Heat the olive oil in a heavy-based pan and gently sauté the onion and celery until soft and translucent. Add the carrots, ginger and tangerine zest, stirring them through. Continue to cook for a couple of minutes before adding the hot stock. Bring to the boil, then reduce the heat to a simmer for about 10 minutes, or until the carrots are soft enough to be easily pierced with a sharp knife.

Allow to cool a little before blending the soup until smooth. Squeeze in half the tangerine juice, stir through and check to see if you need more.

To serve, ladle into bowls and top with a scattering of the cleanse dukkah.

CELERIAC AND UMAMI MUSTARD

Celeriac is often underrated as it is not the most attractive looking vegetable. Celeriac remoulade is one of our favourite dishes and we've brought the flavours of that dish in to this soup.

SERVES 2

2 tbsp olive oil

400g celeriac (about ½ head), cut into 1.5cm cubes

1 tsp umami mustard (page 182)

250ml hot vegetable stock (page 192)

1 tbsp toasted hazelnuts, chopped, to serve (optional)

Heat the oil in a large frying pan and sauté the celeriac until golden brown. Add the umami mustard and stir through the celeriac, then add the hot vegetable stock. Bring to the boil, then reduce the heat to a simmer until the celeriac is cooked and easily pierced with a sharp knife, about 10 minutes.

Allow to cool a little before processing to a smooth consistency in a blender or food processor. Taste to check you have added enough mustard to suit your taste. Scatter over the hazelnuts if you are using them.

CHICKEN CONGEE

White rice is more processed than brown and so it does convert to sugar more quickly. However, we have included it as an option in this Restore recipe as it's so easy on a strained digestion, building it back up to strength. This is a great soup for when you are really struggling with stress or exhaustion or you need to recuperate.

SERVES 2

225g plain white rice (or you could use brown)
750ml chicken stock (pages 187–8)
5cm piece of fresh root ginger, peeled
200g leftover roast chicken, shredded
2 spring onions, thinly sliced on the diagonal
2 tbsp wheat-free tamari soy sauce
1 tbsp toasted sesame oil
2 tsp furikake (or sesame seeds)
handful of fresh coriander leaves, to serve

Add the rice to a large saucepan along with the chicken stock and 1 litre of water. Add the ginger, bring to the boil, then reduce the heat to a very low simmer and cook for about an hour, until the rice has broken down (brown rice will take longer).

To serve, simply ladle the congee into bowls and top with the chicken and spring onions, then drizzle over tamari and toasted sesame oil and scatter with furikake and coriander leaves.

CINNAMON PUMPKIN

Containing both cinnamon and sweet pumpkin, this is a very warming soup for the digestion. It is perfect for the colder months.

SERVES 2

116 kcal

400g pumpkin or
   squash, peeled
   and cubed
1 tbsp groundnut oil
1 tsp ground cinnamon
100g cherry tomatoes
1 tbsp balsamic vinegar
200ml hot vegetable
   stock (page 192)

Preheat the oven to 220°C/425°F/gas mark 7.

In a large bowl, mix the pumpkin with the groundnut oil and cinnamon. Place on a baking tray and roast for 30 minutes, or until cooked through and golden. Check halfway through and give the tray a shake. When the pumpkin pieces are cooked, scatter over the cherry tomatoes and splash with the balsamic vinegar. Return to the oven and turn it off – the residual heat will be enough to burst the tomatoes in about 10 minutes.

Reserve half the tomatoes and blend the remainder in a blender or food processor with the pumpkin and hot vegetable stock until you reach your desired consistency. To serve, ladle the blended soup into bowls and top with the reserved tomatoes.

COD LAKSA

The laksa paste really lifts this soup with the flavours of lemongrass and lime leaves.

SERVES 1

150g cod fillet
2 tsp laksa paste
   (page 180)
1 tsp coconut oil
200ml vegetable stock
   (page 192)
1 pak choi, roughly
   chopped
sea salt flakes and
   freshly ground black
   pepper, to taste

Brush the cod fillet with 1 teaspoon of the laksa paste on the flesh side, season and then fry skin-side down in a little coconut oil until you see the flesh starting to sweat. Flip over, then after a few seconds switch off and leave the fish to sit.

Bring the stock to the boil in a pan, add the remaining teaspoon of laksa paste and stir through. Taste and add more paste if you like. Add the pak choi to the pan and simmer for a minute before removing from the heat. Check for seasoning.

To serve, flake the cod into a bowl and ladle over the broth and vegetables.

CUMIN-ROASTED SWEET POTATO WITH ONION AND POMEGRANATE MOLASSES

We've used cumin here, but you might prefer to substitute it with cinnamon, cardamom or ginger. We have added just a little natural sweetness with the pomegranate molasses.

SERVES 2

2 large sweet potatoes (about 200g), roughly chopped
1 medium onion, peeled and roughly sliced
1 tsp cumin seeds
1 tsp ground turmeric
2 tbsp olive oil
1 tbsp pomegranate molasses
500ml hot vegetable stock (page 192)

Preheat the oven to 200°C/400°F/gas mark 6.

Mix all the ingredients except the stock in a large bowl so the vegetables are evenly coated with the spices, olive oil and molasses.

Roast the vegetables for 15–20 minutes, turning halfway through, until the sweet potatoes are soft and a little caramelised at the edges. Allow to cool slightly before blending the vegetables with the stock to your desired consistency.

GINGER CARROT WITH SPICED COCONUT YOGHURT

The warmth of ginger is balanced by the coconut yoghurt, so simple and always a winning combination.

SERVES 2

FOR THE SOUP

1 tbsp groundnut oil
1/2 onion, chopped
1 tsp freshly grated
    ginger
500g carrots (scrubbed
    if organic, peeled if
    not), roughly chopped
400ml hot vegetable
    stock (page 192)
sea salt flakes and
    freshly ground black
    pepper, to taste

FOR THE YOGHURT

1 tbsp freshly grated or
    desiccated coconut
3 tbsp Greek yoghurt
1 tbsp groundnut oil
6 curry leaves
2 tsp black mustard
    seeds

To make the soup, heat the oil in a saucepan and sauté the onion for about 10 minutes until soft. Add the ginger and stir through for a minute before adding the carrots. Continue to cook, stirring, for a couple of minutes, then add the stock, bring to the boil and reduce to a simmer for 10–15 minutes, or until the carrots can be easily pierced with a sharp knife. Process the soup in a blender or food processor until smooth and taste for seasoning.

To make the coconut yoghurt, mix the grated or desiccated coconut with the Greek yoghurt in a small bowl. Heat the oil in a frying pan and add the curry leaves, allowing them to infuse for a minute before adding the mustard seeds. When the seeds begin to pop, take off the heat, allow to cool a little and then pour over the coconut yoghurt.

To serve the soup, ladle into bowls and spoon over the spiced coconut yoghurt.

JERUSALEM ARTICHOKE AND FENNEL

Jerusalem artichokes are nature's prebiotics, helping to create a fertile environment for your gut flora to flourish.

SERVES 2

314 kcal

300g Jerusalem
   artichokes
a little lemon juice
2 tbsp olive oil
1/2 onion, chopped
1 celery stalk, chopped
1/2 fennel bulb, chopped
350ml hot chicken or
   vegetable stock (pages
   187–8 or 192)
sea salt flakes, to taste
cleanse dukkah (page
   183), to serve
extra virgin olive oil,
   to serve

Scrub the artichokes and soak them for a couple of hours in cold water with a little lemon juice. Drain, then roughly chop them.

Heat the oil in a heavy-based pan and sauté the onion, celery and fennel for 10–15 minutes until soft. Add the artichokes and continue to cook for a couple of minutes before adding the hot stock. Bring to the boil, then reduce the heat to a simmer and cook for 10–15 minutes, or until the artichokes are soft. Whiz in a blender or food processor until smooth, then taste for seasoning.

To serve, ladle into bowls and scatter with cleanse dukkah and a drizzle of extra virgin olive oil.

LENTILS, SEASONAL GREENS AND GINGER CARROT COLESLAW

To make Puy lentils really tasty, we cook them as if they were in a risotto. They are a great vegetarian source of protein.

SERVES 2

343 kcal

1 tbsp olive oil
1/2 onion, peeled and
   finely chopped
100g Puy lentils
400ml hot vegetable
   stock (page 192)
1 large or 2 small carrots
   (washed and scrubbed
   if organic, peeled if
   not), grated
1/2 tsp freshly grated
   ginger
100g winter or spring
   greens
2 egg yolks, in the shell

Heat the oil in a frying pan or heavy-based saucepan and soften the onion for 8–10 minutes. Add the Puy lentils and stir through the onion for a minute before adding the hot vegetable stock. Simmer for about 30 minutes until cooked but still with a little bite.

Stir the carrots and ginger together. Steam the greens for a few minutes until cooked but still a little crunchy.

To serve, divide the lentils and broth between two bowls and top with the carrot and greens. Carefully separate the egg yolks from the whites, keeping the yolk in one half of the shell to serve in the bowl. When you eat the soup, stir the yolk through the lentils and discard the shell.

MAGIC SOUP

This soup includes a mix of spices that stoke the digestive fire back to strength.

SERVES 2

343 kcal

250g yellow split peas, rinsed
¹/₄ tsp cayenne pepper
¹/₂ tsp ground turmeric
1 tbsp coconut oil
1 onion, sliced
¹/₂ tsp ground cinnamon
¹/₂ tsp ground ginger
¹/₂ tsp garam masala
180g baby spinach
2 tbsp toasted mixed seeds (pumpkin, sesame, hemp, flax), to serve

Put the split peas in a saucepan with 1 litre of water, the cayenne pepper and turmeric, and bring to the boil. Reduce the heat to a simmer and cook gently for about 1 hour, or until the split peas are soft and broken up. Remove half the split peas and process to a smooth consistency in a blender or food processor, then return them to the pan and stir through the reserved split peas.

Heat the coconut oil in a large frying pan, add the onion and cook gently for about 10 minutes, until soft. Add the spices and continue to cook until the aromas are released. Add the spinach to the pan and stir through to wilt.

Reheat the split pea soup, divide between two serving bowls, top with the spiced spinach and onions and scatter over the toasted mixed seeds.

ROASTED BUCKWHEAT WITH ACHARI SPICES AND EXOTIC MUSHROOMS

Mushrooms such as shiitake, enoki, crimini and oyster contain properties that stimulate the immune system.

SERVES 2

1 onion, finely chopped
1 tbsp groundnut oil
1/2 tsp cumin seeds
1/2 tsp fennel seeds
1/2 tsp mustard seeds
1/2 tsp ground turmeric
    (or 1/4 fresh turmeric,
    grated)
100g roasted buckwheat
400ml hot vegetable
    stock (page 192)
100g exotic mushrooms
    (such as shiitake,
    golden enoki, white
    enoki, shimeji)
1 tbsp coconut oil,
    melted

Sauté the onion in the groundnut oil in a heavy-based pan. After a few minutes, add the cumin, fennel and mustard seeds and turmeric. Stir and allow the aromas to be released from the spices. Stir in the buckwheat, followed by some hot vegetable stock – enough to cover the buckwheat. Cook for about 15 minutes or until tender.

Meanwhile, sauté a mixture of exotic mushrooms in a little coconut oil.

To serve, ladle the buckwheat broth into bowls and top with the mushrooms.

SPROUTED SOUP

It's a good idea to make a large pot of this soup as it's so good for you and tastes pretty surprising, considering it's really just beans and spices with an added helping of nutritional live sprouts on top.

SERVES 2

80g dried aduki beans,
   soaked for 48 hours
   (change the water 3
   times daily) and rinsed
500ml hot vegetable
   stock (page 192)
1 tsp ground turmeric
2 tbsp light sesame oil
   (or olive oil)
1 tsp cleanse spice mix
   (page 183)
2 tbsp radish or alfalfa
   sprouts, to serve
kefir or natural yoghurt,
   to serve

Add the beans to a saucepan along with the hot vegetable stock and turmeric. Bring to the boil, then gently simmer until the beans have slightly broken down into a thick soup, about 1 ½ hours.

Meanwhile, heat the oil in a small non-stick frying pan and when hot add the cleanse spice mix. When the spices begin to release their aroma, take the pan off the heat, and once cooled a little, add them to the soup as it's cooking and give it a good stir.

Serve the soup with a handful of sprouted seeds for extra goodness and a spoonful of kefir or natural yoghurt.

WHITE KIMCHI

Our take on 'cabbage soup' but a little more interesting with the probiotic power of fermented kimchi and miso broth. Do add some buckwheat soba noodles if you want to make it more substantial.

SERVES 1

200ml very hot white miso stock

2 heaped tbsp kimchi (page 184)

50g fresh silken tofu, cubed

1 spring onion, thinly sliced, to serve

1 tsp white sesame seeds, to serve

Heat the miso stock. In a bowl, arrange the kimchi and the tofu then pour over the very hot stock. Scatter over the sliced spring onion and the sesame seeds to serve.

RENEW

BARLEY BONE BROTH

This soup may give you powers! Bone broths, like bone marrow, is real 'essence' food; a little goes a long way.

SERVES 2

1 tbsp groundnut oil
1 leek, thinly sliced
2 carrots, chopped
160g cooked barley
400ml hot bone broth
    (page 191)
freshly ground black
    pepper, to taste

Heat the oil in a heavy-based pan and add the leek. Gently sauté until soft, then add the carrots and continue to cook for a few minutes. Add the cooked barley and stir through the vegetables. Pour over the hot bone broth, bring to the boil and then reduce the heat to a simmer for a few more minutes until the carrot is cooked but still has a little bite.

Season with plenty of freshly ground black pepper and serve.

BEETROOT AND CARAWAY

Caraway seeds are said to be beneficial for digestive problems and add a lovely flavour to the intensity of the beetroot.

SERVES 2 136 kcal

4 large or 6 small
   whole beetroot
2 tbsp apple cider
   vinegar
1 tsp caraway seeds
300–400ml hot
   vegetable stock
   (page 192)
2 tbsp chopped fresh dill
sea salt flakes and
   freshly ground black
   pepper, to taste
natural yoghurt, to serve

Preheat the oven to 200°C/400°F/gas mark 6.

Wash the beetroot and cut off all but 2.5cm of the stalks. Place in a roasting tray and add enough water to come about halfway up the sides, plus the vinegar. Scatter over the caraway seeds, cover the tray with foil and bake in the oven until soft, about 45 minutes.

Remove from the oven, take off the foil, remove the beetroot from the cooking liquid and allow to cool, then rub off the skins with kitchen paper. Roughly chop the beetroot, then blend with the stock and dill to reach the consistency you prefer. Check for seasoning.

Serve warm or cold with a little natural yoghurt.

CAULIFLOWER, GARLIC AND WALNUT CRUMB

As part of the cruciferous family, cauliflower is supportive of the body's own detoxification system and contains both antioxidant and anti-inflammatory properties. Garlic is naturally anti-inflammatory too, while walnuts are considered in Chinese medicine to support our 'essence'.

SERVES 2

256 kcal

300ml almond milk
3 garlic cloves
1/2 medium cauliflower (500g), cut into florets
sea salt and freshly ground black pepper, to taste
20g walnuts, to serve
drizzle of rosemary infused oil, to serve (page 186)

Bring the almond milk almost to the boil in a pan, add the whole garlic cloves and simmer for 10 minutes. Remove the garlic and add the cauliflower florets, continuing to simmer until they are tender and cooked, 7–10 minutes. Allow the soup to cool a little before blending in a blender or food processor until smooth. Check for seasoning.

Wrap the walnuts in a tea towel and bash with a rolling pin, then shake them through a large sieve to remove the skins.

To serve, ladle the soup into bowls, drizzle over a swirl of rosemary oil and scatter over the walnut crumbs.

CHICKEN AND NETTLE TOPS

Nettle soup is traditionally made in the spring and makes a fresh change from eating lots of preserved foods all winter. We might have access to fresh foods all year round now but spring still feels like the perfect time to lighten things up and have a good cleanse, so keep this recipe on hand for when you see fresh young nettles begin to appear. You can also add nettles to the lemon, chicken and mint soup (page 112) when in season.

SERVES 1

274 kcal

150ml chicken stock
(pages 187–8)
100g leftover chicken,
shredded
40g nettle tops
2 tbsp wheat-free tamari
soy sauce

Bring the chicken stock to the boil in a pan. Reduce the heat to a simmer and add the chicken. After a couple of minutes add the nettle tops and simmer until wilted, just a minute or so.

Add the tamari sauce and taste for seasoning, before serving straightaway.

FENNEL-CRUSTED SALMON WITH GINGER CHINESE CABBAGE

Seeds such as fennel, cumin or coriander and citrus zests and peels are the perfect way to add extra layers of taste, texture and bonus nutrition to our cooking.

SERVES 2

311 kcal

1 tsp fennel seeds
zest of 1 lime
1 tsp coconut oil
1 large or 2 small salmon
    fillets
1 tsp Dijon or umami
    mustard (page 182)
300ml vegetable stock
    (page 192)
thumb-sized piece of
    fresh ginger, thickly
    sliced
1 small Chinese cabbage
    (or half a large),
    thickly sliced

Preheat the oven to 150°C/300°F/gas mark 2.

Scatter the fennel seeds and lime zest over a baking sheet and dry in the oven for 10 minutes. Transfer to a pestle and mortar and crush the seeds. Turn up the oven to 220°C/425°F/gas mark 7.

Heat a little coconut oil in a hot pan and fry the salmon fillet skin side down for about 3 minutes to crisp the skin. Take off the heat and spread a little mustard on each fillet, then scatter with the fennel and lime mix. Cook for another 5 minutes in the oven (longer if you prefer salmon cooked all the way through).

For the ginger-braised cabbage, put the vegetable stock and ginger slices into a large shallow saucepan along with the Chinese cabbage. Bring to the boil then reduce the heat to a gentle simmer for about 10 minutes until the cabbage is cooked but still has a nice bite to it.

To serve, place the cabbage in bowls and ladle over the broth. Flake the salmon and divide between the bowls.

HARISSA BROTH WITH AUBERGINE AND QUINOA

This is a deep and nourishing soup which builds you up from your foundations. In Chinese medicine, it is said aubergine will nourish your blood and quinoa your qi or vitality.

SERVES 2

194 kcal

1 aubergine, sliced into 4cm rounds
20ml olive oil
sea salt flakes, to taste
250ml vegetable stock (page 192)
1 tsp rose harissa
100g black quinoa (or white)
saffron yoghurt (page 185), to serve

Preheat the oven to 240°C/475°F/gas mark 9.

Place the aubergine rounds in a mixing bowl and drizzle over the olive oil, combining thoroughly so that all the aubergine rounds are covered. Season with sea salt flakes. Spread out the aubergine in a roasting tray and roast in the oven for 10–15 minutes until golden, turning halfway through.

Meanwhile, bring the stock to the boil in a pan and add the harissa and quinoa. Reduce the heat to a simmer and cook for 8 minutes. Turn off the heat and allow to rest so the quinoa puffs.

Set aside 4 slices of aubergine then quarter the remaining slices, adding the quarters to the quinoa and harissa broth. Stir in and let this sit.

To serve, heat the soup and divide between two bowls. Set the aubergine rounds on top and add saffron yoghurt over the soup using a slotted spoon.

GREEN PHO

*A vibrant soup full of Eastern anti-oxidant and anti-inflammatory goodness.
Do add either some fresh organic tofu or brown rice noodles to this soup if
you'd like to make it more substantial.*

SERVES 1

1 tsp crushed fresh
   ginger
$1/_2$ fresh red chilli,
   deseeded and finely
   sliced
2 spring onions, finely
   sliced
100g tat soi, or other
   Asian greens, stalks
   chopped
a few lime or Thai
   basil leaves (or use
   coriander), plus
   extra to serve
handful of beansprouts
1 lime wedge
250ml hot seaweed
   broth (page 189)

The night before you want to eat this soup,
put all the ingredients except the lime and
stock into a jar and mix well to combine.

To serve, simply pour the hot vegetable
stock into the jar, squeeze over the lime and
stir to combine.

MUSSELS AND LEEK

Often shellfish will be left out of a cleanse because they may be high in heavy metals, picked up from the ocean floor. On the other hand, they are a rich source of many energising vitamins and minerals. We go for a varied diet and so are happy to include shellfish on occasion.

SERVES 2

372 kcal

1kg mussels, cleaned and debearded
1 tbsp coconut oil
1/2 onion, finely chopped
1/2 celery stalk, finely chopped
1 leek, finely chopped
50ml sake (optional)
200ml vegetable stock (page 192)

Check through the mussels, discarding any open ones that don't close when tapped firmly on the work surface.

Heat the oil in a heavy-based saucepan, add the onion and celery and cook gently for 5 minutes, then add the leek and continue to soften for 10 minutes. Add the sake, if using, and vegetable stock, then add the mussels. Give everything a good stir, cover with a lid and then remove from the heat with the lid still on so the mussels cook in the residual heat. The mussels will open once cooked.

To serve, simply divide the mussels and leek broth between bowls. Remove and discard any mussels that haven't opened. Treat yourself to a piece of sourdough to mop up the broth with!

RAW SOUP

This is perfect for a warm, sunny day. The cucumber is cooling while the avocado satisfies. The kefir nourishes your gut flora while the kale/spinach adds a burst of antioxidants.

SERVES 2

1 medium ripe
   Hass avocado
1/2 medium cucumber,
   roughly chopped
handful of baby spinach
   or kale leaves
zest and juice of 1/2 lime
   (plus more juice
   to taste)
75ml natural yoghurt
   or kefir
3 ice cubes
2 spring onions,
   finely chopped
1 tbsp finely chopped
   coriander
sea salt and freshly
   ground black pepper,
   to taste

Whiz all the ingredients except the spring onions and coriander in a food processor or blender until smooth. Add a little cold water if the soup seems too thick. Taste for lime and seasoning. Transfer to the refrigerator to chill before serving.

Combine the spring onions, lime zest and coriander to make a salsa. Serve the chilled soup with a dollop of salsa on top.

CRAB, FENNEL AND TURMERIC CONGEE

Congee is simply rice slow-cooked in much larger quantities of water than we are often used to. The rice is cooked until it breaks down and turns the liquid thick and creamy. It has a mild, sweet flavour and is incredibly easy on the digestion, which makes it very nourishing.

SERVES 2

316 kcal

1 cup short, medium or long grain rice (or brown, not basmati), rinsed

4 cups chicken or vegetable stock (optional)

$1/4$ tsp grated fresh turmeric or 1 tsp ground turmeric

1 tbsp toasted sesame oil

100g white crab meat

1 small raw fennel bulb, thinly sliced

3 spring onions, thinly sliced

a few thin slices of pickled ginger

2 tsp furikake (or sesame seeds)

The easiest way to make congee is on the hob. Add the rice to a heavy-based saucepan along with the stock, 3 cups of water and the turmeric.

Bring the rice to an easy boil and then reduce to a low simmer for 30–90 minutes, depending on the consistency you prefer. Stir occasionally to prevent the rice sticking to the bottom of the pan. The longer you can wait, the better!

Serve the congee in deep bowls and drizzle a little sesame oil over. Scatter over the fresh crab meat, fennel slices and spring onions. Top with the ginger and furikake (or sesame seeds).

RED LENTIL AND TAMARIND

We love to experiment with different versions of dal and this combination of fibre-rich red lentils with tamarind is a new favourite.

SERVES 2

100g dried red lentils, rinsed
500ml vegetable stock (page 192)
1 tsp ground turmeric
1 tsp garam masala
1 tbsp tamarind paste
3cm piece of fresh root ginger, peeled and grated
1 tbsp tomato paste
120g cooked brown rice
2 tbsp natural yoghurt or kefir
fresh coriander leaves, to serve

Add the lentils to a heavy-based pan and add the stock, turmeric, garam masala, tamarind paste and ginger. Bring to the boil, then reduce the heat and simmer until the lentils are soft, about 20 minutes, adding the tomato paste about halfway through.

Stir through the brown rice to heat well, then serve immediately with a spoonful of natural yoghurt or kefir and some fresh coriander leaves scattered over.

ROAST CHICKPEA

Chickpeas and paprika were made to go together. Apparently, chickpeas may even help to trigger feelings of satiety, very useful when we are retraining our appetite after the holidays.

SERVES 2

188 kcal

200g dried chickpeas, soaked in water for 24 hours
1 bay leaf
1 garlic clove, smashed
1 tsp Turkish chilli (Aleppo pepper or Turkish paprika)
1 tsp smoked paprika
1 tsp allspice
1 tbsp tomato paste
1 tbsp honey
1 red chilli, deseeded and sliced
dash of cider vinegar
200ml hot vegetable stock (page 192)
bunch of fresh coriander, chopped, to serve
natural yoghurt or kefir, to serve

Drain and rinse the chickpeas well and add to a pan, cover with plenty of water, and add the bay leaf and the garlic. Bring to the boil, then reduce the heat to a simmer and cook for 1 hour.

Preheat the oven to 220°C/425°F/gas mark 7. Remove the bay leaf, drain the chickpeas and add them to a mixing bowl along with all the dried spices, tomato paste, honey and chilli and mix well. Spread over a baking tray, add a dash of cider vinegar and roast in the oven for 10–15 minutes.

Blend the roasted chickpeas with the hot stock (or if you prefer, keep them whole or half of them whole) in a blender or food processor, and garnish with plenty of chopped coriander and a spoonful of natural yoghurt or kefir.

SESAME CHICKEN

In Chinese medicine it is said we deplete our 'essence' through consuming too many stimulants and not enough minerals, but we can help to redress the balance through good rest, relaxation and a nourishing diet that includes nutrient-dense foods such as chicken, seaweed, nettles and sesame seeds.

SERVES 2

362 kcal

- 80g buckwheat or brown rice noodles
- 1 tsp groundnut oil
- 1 tsp light sesame oil
- 5cm piece of fresh root ginger, peeled and finely sliced into matchsticks
- 4 large or 6 small shiitake mushrooms (fresh or soaked if dried)
- 2 boneless chicken breasts, cut into bite-size pieces (or leftover chicken)
- 1 tbsp brown rice vinegar
- 400ml chicken stock (pages 187–8)
- 1 tsp toasted sesame oil
- 1 tsp fish sauce
- 1 tbsp wheat-free tamari soy sauce
- 2 spring onions, thinly sliced on the diagonal
- 2 tsp furikake or sesame seeds (black or white)

Bring a pan of water to the boil and add the noodles. Bring back to the boil and cook for 3–5 minutes (check the packet for timings). Drain the noodles, then rinse under cold water and drain again.

Heat the groundnut and sesame oils in a wok over a high heat and when the oil starts to smoke, add the ginger and shiitake mushrooms and stir-fry for a few seconds before adding the chicken. Continue to stir-fry until the chicken has browned a little and then add the brown rice vinegar to deglaze the wok. Add the stock, sesame oil, fish sauce and tamari, bring to the boil, then reduce the heat and simmer for 10 minutes.

To serve, place the cooked noodles into bowls and ladle the soup over. Scatter over the spring onions and furikake or sesame seeds.

SOPA DE QUINOA

As a seed, rather than a grain, quinoa contains a surprising amount of protein. We love the black and red varieties that are more readily available now.

SERVES 2

80g red quinoa
(or white)
300ml vegetable stock
(page 192)
2 tbsp raw pistachios
good handful of basil
leaves
1 tbsp umami mustard
(page 182)
4 tbsp extra virgin
olive oil
150g green beans
sea salt flakes, to taste
50g pea shoots, to serve

Add the quinoa and vegetable stock to a pan and bring to the boil. Reduce the heat to a simmer and cook for about 15 minutes or until the quinoa is cooked but still has a little bite.

Meanwhile, toast the pistachio nuts for a minute in a dry frying pan before blending them with the basil and mustard in a food processor, slowly adding the olive oil with the motor running to form a smooth pesto.

Steam or boil the green beans until al dente and add to the quinoa broth. Taste for seasoning.

To serve, ladle the broth into bowls and add a spoonful of the pistachio pesto, then scatter over the pea shoots.

SQUASH AND ALMOND BUTTER

Not only do almonds contain heart-healthy monounsaturated fats but they have been shown to help decrease blood sugar imbalances after eating, so are good to eat as part of a meal, not only as a snack.

SERVES 2
376 kcal

1 tbsp groundnut oil
1 small or ¹/₂ large onion, peeled and sliced
¹/₂ butternut squash, peeled and chopped into cubes
1 carrot (scrubbed if organic, peeled if not), chopped into cubes
500ml hot vegetable or chicken stock (pages 192 or 187–8)
2 tbsp crunchy almond butter
1 tsp chopped almonds, to serve
Greek yoghurt or kefir, to serve (optional)

Heat the oil in a heavy-based pan, add the onion, and sauté for about 10 minutes until soft and translucent. Add the squash and carrot and continue to sauté for a few minutes, stirring occasionally.

Add the hot stock and the almond butter, bring to the boil, then reduce the heat to a simmer and cook gently for 15–20 minutes, or until the vegetables are tender. Allow to cool a little before processing in a blender to make a smooth soup.

Serve scattered with chopped almonds and a swirl of Greek yoghurt or kefir, if you like.

WATERCRESS, FLAX AND TOFU

We gave ourselves the challenge of making a creamy watercress soup
without potatoes or cream, and tofu provided the answer.

SERVES 2
248 kcal

400ml chicken or
   vegetable stock
   (pages 187–8 or 192)
80g watercress, rinsed
80g spinach, rinsed
2 tbsp ground flaxseeds
50g fresh tofu, cubed
sea salt and freshly
   ground black pepper,
   to taste
natural yoghurt, to serve
2 tsp toasted hemp
   seeds, to serve

In a saucepan, bring the stock to the boil.
Add the watercress and spinach to allow
them to wilt in the heat of the pan, then take
the pan off the heat. After a couple of
minutes, add the ground flaxseeds and tofu
and blend the soup in a blender or food
processor. Check for seasoning, before
serving topped with natural yoghurt and
toasted hemp seeds.

WILD RICE, EDAMAME AND RAINBOW CHARD

This soup is brimming with nutrients from the dark leafy greens and seaweeds.

SERVES 2

50g wild rice, rinsed
   thoroughly
50g edamame beans,
   popped
50g samphire
300ml seaweed broth
   (page 189)
100g rainbow chard,
   washed
cleanse dukkah (page
   183), to serve

Tip the rice into a pan and cover with plenty of water, then bring to the boil. Reduce the heat and simmer for about 40 minutes, or until the rice is cooked – wild rice takes longer than white rice. Drain.

In another pan of simmering water, blanch the edamame and samphire for a couple of minutes. Drain.

Bring the seaweed broth to the boil in another pan, and stir through the rice and all the vegetables. Remove from the heat.

Divide the soup between two bowls and scatter over some cleanse dukkah to serve.

WINTER CHICKEN

Rainbow chard is a wonderful vegetable that brings a vibrant colour to dishes throughout the year. It is so robust that it will happily grow during the colder months.

SERVES 2

1 tbsp groundnut oil
1 leek, finely sliced
100g rainbow chard, shredded
200g cooked chicken, shredded
400ml hot chicken stock (pages 187–8)
2 tbsp Greek yoghurt, to serve
1 tbsp hazelnuts, halved and toasted, to serve
sea salt and freshly ground black pepper, to taste

Heat the oil in a heavy-based pan and sauté the leek until soft. Add the chard and continue to cook for a couple of minutes before adding the chicken followed by the hot stock. Bring to the boil and then reduce the heat to a simmer and cook until the chard is cooked – a few minutes. Check for seasoning then ladle into bowls, and top with a spoonful of Greek yoghurt and some toasted hazelnuts.

SOUP JARS

This is a great way to take your soup to work; just add hot water, mix it up and devour!

The basis of the soup jar concept is to have your noodles or grain at the bottom of a sealable jar, topped with layers of a flavour paste, some protein and a few veggies. We've included four ideas here, each of which serve 1 person, to get you started, but feel free to personalise your soups with your favourite ingredients. Layer up!

KIMCHI MISO TOFU

100g cooked buckwheat noodles
1 tsp white miso paste, loosened in a little hot water
2 tbsp white kimchi (page 141)
50g fresh tofu, cubed

COCONUT PRAWN

100g cooked brown rice noodles
1 tsp Thai paste (page 181)
100g prawns, cooked in a little coconut oil
1 small carrot, grated
handful of alfalfa, radish or broccoli sprouts

SHIITAKE SEAWEED MISO

50g soaked seaweed spaghetti (soaked weight)
1 tsp white miso paste, loosened in a little hot water
2–3 shiitake mushrooms, soaked and sliced
50g smoked tofu, cubed

CHICKEN AND BABY KALE LAKSA

60g cooked buckwheat noodles
1 tsp laksa paste (page 180)
80g leftover roast chicken
50g baby kale or baby spinach

CHAPTER 7:
CLEANSE-ENHANCING RECIPES

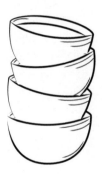

All calorie counts are per single serving.

OVERNIGHT OATS

It isn't always easy to have a good breakfast when you're rushing to work or organising the children instead of making time to look after yourself. This recipe for overnight oats is so versatile that you can add all kinds of toppings, and all you need to do is let the oats soften while you sleep, so they'll be ready for you first thing. Soaking oats makes them even easier to digest, which is good news when you're trying to give your body a chance to rest and restore.

These will keep in the refrigerator in an airtight container for three days, so you can make plenty ahead of time.

SERVES 1   221 kcal

50g rolled oats (use
    gluten-free if you are
    intolerant)
1 tsp flaxseeds
1 tsp chia seeds
1 tsp sesame seeds
pinch of ground
    cinnamon
150ml almond or coconut
    milk (or coconut water,
    if you prefer)
couple of drops of
    vanilla extract

Combine all the dry ingredients and then add your liquid of choice along with the vanilla extract, stirring thoroughly. Transfer to a glass jar with an airtight lid and set in the fridge. The oats will be ready within a few hours.

CLOVE-SPICED APPLE

Heat your overnight oats with a little more water or nut milk in a pan. Chop an apple into cubes, heat a little coconut oil in a frying pan and add about 6 cloves. Once the cloves release their aroma, remove them from the oil and add the apple cubes. Now chop a few skin-on almonds and add to the apples. Once the apples have caramelised a little, serve the apples and almonds on top of the oats.

BIRCHER

Bircher muesli is served cold, so it's super easy to prepare first thing. When you are ready to serve the overnight oats, stir in the juice of half a lime, a few chopped hazelnuts, a chopped apple or pear and a couple of heaped spoonfuls of natural yoghurt, if you like.

BERRY COMPOTE

Heat 50g frozen berries (blueberries, raspberries, blackberries) in a small pan with a little water and honey until they begin to break down and reduce to form a lovely compote. You can keep this in the refrigerator in an airtight jar for up to a week.

To serve with the overnight oats, heat the oats in a pan with a little more of your preferred milk and top with the compote and a spoonful of natural yoghurt, if you like.

EGG DROP SOUP WITH NORI

When you have a little extra time for breakfast this is a lovely way to enjoy eggs without the usual slice of toast. Many Asian cultures start the day with broth or soup rather than sweet cereals or bakery foods.

SERVES 1

260 kcal

1 tsp white miso paste or sachet miso soup
1 tsp nori flakes
1 egg, beaten
1 spring onion, finely sliced
1 tsp sesame oil
sea salt and freshly ground black pepper, to taste

Place the miso paste in a saucepan, add about 300ml of just-boiled water (or according to the instructions on the packet) and stir thoroughly to dissolve. Bring the miso to a simmer. Add the nori flakes and stir through. Very slowly pour the egg into the soup in a thin stream, stirring gently, to create ribbons as the egg cooks.

Remove from the heat and taste for seasoning. Serve scattered with spring onion and with a little sesame oil drizzled over.

MISO BREAKFAST BROTH

This is another savoury breakfast option to fire up your energy in the morning.

SERVES 1

148 kcal

20g quinoa
40g buckwheat
$1/2$ tsp brown miso paste
a few strips of wakame
    seaweed, soaked and
    cut into 2cm pieces
40g fresh tofu, cubed
$1/2$ tsp black (or white)
    sesame seeds

Bring a pan of water to the boil and cook the quinoa and buckwheat according to the packet instructions. Drain the grains and set aside.

In the meantime, add the miso paste to about 300ml of just-boiled water (or according to the instructions on the packet) and stir thoroughly to dissolve.

To serve, add the buckwheat, seaweed and tofu to the miso and scatter over the sesame seeds.

You can make this the night before; make up the broth but don't add the tofu, then in the morning heat up the miso, add the seaweed and buckwheat and add the tofu just before serving.

SMOOTHIES

The great thing about whizzing up a smoothie is that you can pack it with healthy ingredients and take it out with you. Berries are our favourite fruits and so we love to combine them with kefir for a boost as in the smoothie below. The almond chia and avocado nuts smoothies are particularly good for vegetarians or if you are having a meat-free day as they contain both protein and good fats.

BERRY KEFIR BOOSTER

Kefir is fermented and contains masses of beneficial bacteria. It's like yoghurt, so if you can't find it, use live natural yoghurt instead.

SERVES 1

146 kcal

1 cup frozen blueberries
100ml kefir
a little unsweetened
    almond milk
couple of drops of
    vanilla extract
ground flaxseeds
    or vitality powder
    (optional)

Blitz together the frozen blueberries, the kefir and the unsweetened almond milk. Add vanilla extract for a little extra sweetness. You can also add some ground flaxseeds or a natural vitality powder.

ALMOND CHIA

SERVES 1 312 kcal

1 tbsp almond butter
2 tbsp natural yoghurt
1 tbsp soaked chia
  seeds (1 tsp dry seeds
  soaked in 4 tbsp water
  overnight)
$^1/_2$ frozen banana
  or 3 tbsp frozen
  blueberries
150ml coconut milk

Blend all the ingredients together until smooth.

AVOCADO NUTS

SERVES 2

271
kcal

Blend all the ingredients together until well combined and refrigerate before serving.

1 avocado
250ml almond milk
1 tbsp almond butter
1 tsp flaxseed oil
1 tsp agave syrup
1 tsp grated fresh ginger

NOURISH BITES

These are perfect to have on hand for when you need a bit of nourishment and if you weren't careful you'd find yourself grabbing a chocolate bar instead. They are also great for days when you are working out.

MAKES 10

70g almonds

30g hemp seeds

120g dried apple

1 tsp spirulina

1 tsp acai powder

2 tbsp coconut oil

30g shredded coconut

2 tbsp runny honey

1 tbsp sesame seeds,
   for rolling

Place all the ingredients, except the sesame seeds, into a food processor and blend to a paste. Roll into balls and coat with the sesame seeds. Store in the fridge in an airtight container for up to 5 days.

KALE CRISPS

Kate loves crisps, and these crunchy bites of kale satisfy even her cravings..

SERVES 4

56
kcal

Preheat the oven to 120°C/275°F/gas mark 1.

Toss the shredded kale with the olive oil and a good pinch of salt. Spread out in an even layer over an oven tray and bake for about 20 minutes, turning halfway through, until crispy. Add the pumpkin seeds for the last 5 minutes to toast.

100g kale, shredded
1 tbsp olive oil
1 tbsp pumpkin seeds
sea salt flakes

TURMERIC AND BLACK PEPPER OATCAKES

You can add lots of different flavours to homemade oatcakes, such as dried herbs, paprika and other spices. One of our favourite combinations is turmeric and black pepper, and these oatcakes make the perfect accompaniment to all our vegetarian soups.

MAKES ABOUT 20 OATCAKES

51 kcal

250g porridge oats
1 tbsp olive oil
$1/_4$ tsp ground turmeric
good pinch freshly
   ground black pepper
$1/_4$ tsp sea salt

Preheat the oven to 180°C/350°F/gas mark 4.

Put the oats in a large bowl, add the olive oil, turmeric, pepper and salt and mix.

Fill a jug with half boiled, half cool water and add enough of it to the oats to make them sticky enough to form a ball that binds together. If you add too much water, just add some more oats. Roll out the ball into a large thin, square shape, then score into small, cracker-size squares and use a spatula to lift the pieces onto a baking tray.

Bake until golden, for 20–30 minutes, depending on thickness.

DRINKS

Drinking plenty of water throughout the day is one of the best things you can do for your digestion. The only time when it is best not to drink a lot of water is while you are eating, so as not to flood the digestive system at the same time as it is handling food.

First thing in the morning, sip hot water with a squeeze of lemon. You can add some fresh mint, too.

The best cleansing teas include:

- Fennel
- Nettle
- Dandelion
- Green
- Fresh mint

Green tea is a powerful antioxidant and activates enzymes in the liver that help to eliminate toxins from the body. It needs to be steeped for 5-10 minutes to release its catechins and is best drunk within the hour.

If you are feeling brave, drink a glass of water each day with a capful of apple cider vinegar in it. Look out for kombucha in your local natural food store. It is a fermented drink made with beneficial bacteria and has a tangy taste that Kate loves.

Naturally flavoured waters:

- Strips of cucumber and scrunched mint leaves
- Lemon and lime

Naturally flavoured coconut water:

Coconut water is packed with potassium and is naturally isotonic, helping your body to rehydrate itself, particularly after exercise. Add:

- Melon juice
- Cucumber and mint

And for a hot, health-boosting drink add a little turmeric, lemon juice, fresh ginger and honey to hot water.

PASTES, CHUTNEYS AND MAKE-AHEAD GARNISHES

SPROUTS

Traditional cultures that consume grains regularly sprout the grains to make them more digestible. Sprouting breaks down the anti-nutrients found in grains making the nutrients in the grain more bioavailable. The sprouting process itself boosts the nutrient profile of the grain – increases its vitamin content – and can help with the bloating and pain that some people experience from beans, pulses or grains. We will often sprout mung beans for just a couple of days before making kitchari soup (page 111) and love to add different sprouts to soups and salads as a garnish.

What you can sprout:

- Aduki beans
- Alfalfa seeds
- Barley grains
- Broccoli seeds
- Celery seeds
- Chica seeds
- Chickpeas
- Green peas
- Lentils
- Mung beans
- Pumpkin seeds
- Radish seeds
- Sesame seeds
- Spelt grains
- Sunflower seeds

How to sprout:

Soak your chosen seeds overnight in a bowl of water. In the morning, drain the seeds and rinse them with fresh water once or twice. Place the seeds in a sprouting jar without any water and set it on its side. Screw on the lid with the mesh insert to allow the sprouts to breathe. Every morning and night rinse the sprouts in the jar with fresh water, drain, and set the jar on its side again. The seeds should be sprouting within 1–4 days.

LAKSA PASTE

You can store this homemade laksa paste in an airtight container in the fridge, where it will keep for up to 1 month. Add vegetable or chicken stock and some fish or chicken to make a meal, or simply serve it with brown rice or noodles.

2 tbsp coriander seeds

2 tbsp cumin seeds

8 star anise

50g red chilli, deseeded and chopped

100g piece of fresh root ginger, peeled and roughly chopped

1 tsp galangal

15 kaffir lime leaves

7 lemongrass stalks

sesame oil, to blend

(26 kcal)

Heat a small non-stick frying pan and dry-fry the coriander, cumin and star anise until they just begin to release their aromas. Tip out of the pan onto a plate to cool for a couple of minutes, then grind in a spice grinder or pestle and mortar.

Place the ground spices in a food processor along with the remaining paste ingredients, adding just enough sesame oil to help it blend to a smooth, but not runny, paste.

THAI PASTE

You can store this homemade paste in an airtight container in the fridge, where it will keep for up to 1 month.

2 green chillies, finely chopped

(16 kcal)

2 lemongrass stalks, finely chopped

4cm piece of fresh root ginger, peeled and grated

zest and juice of 2 limes

12 kaffir lime leaves

1 tsp coriander seeds

1 tsp cumin seeds

Put all the paste ingredients in a pestle and mortar or food processor and blend until smooth.

CELERIAC AND
UMAMI MUSTARD PASTE

We found this sensational mustard called 'Anarchy in a Jar' when we were visiting Brooklyn; it has the most incredible list of ingredients and we use it as a basis for several soups in this book.

You can make this mustard a few days ahead of when you want to use it, as it will keep in an airtight container in the refrigerator for one month.

100g yellow mustard seeds (or brown if you prefer hotter mustard)

14 kcal

150ml cider vinegar
100ml matcha green tea (or water), cooled
¹/₄ tsp nori flakes
1 tbsp runny honey
¹/₂ tsp finely grated fresh ginger
¹/₄ tsp smoked paprika
¹/₄ tsp sea salt flakes

Soak the mustard seeds in the cider vinegar and cold matcha green tea for 48 hours in a jar with the lid off. After this time, pour the seeds and any remaining liquid into a food processor along with the nori flakes, honey, ginger, paprika and salt and blend to a paste.

CLEANSE SPICE MIX

1 tsp black
  mustard seeds
1 tsp cumin seeds
1 tsp fennel seeds
1 tsp black onion seeds

12
kcal

Simply mix all the seeds together and keep in an airtight jar in a cool, dry place.

CLEANSE DUKKAH

1 tbsp sesame seeds
1 tbsp pumpkin seeds
1 tbsp hemp seeds
$\frac{1}{2}$ tsp nori flakes
$\frac{1}{4}$ tsp ground turmeric

17
kcal

Mix all the ingredients together and keep in an airtight jar in a cool, dry place.

KIMCHI

This recipe is adapted from a 'white kimchi' recipe we came across in Bon Appetit and love. It is a cross between Korean kimchi and sauerkraut.

4cm piece fresh root ginger, peeled

(42 kcal)

3 garlic cloves, peeled

2 tbsp sea salt

1 white cabbage (approx 500g), shredded

½ daikon, peeled and thinly sliced

4 spring onions, thinly sliced

Process the ginger, garlic and salt to a paste.

Put the paste in a large bowl along with all the vegetables, and massage with your hands until thoroughly combined and the cabbage begins to release its own juices. As you continue, more liquid will be released until there is enough to cover the cabbage when it is pressed down.

Transfer the cabbage and all the liquid to a preserving jar. You need to put weight on the cabbage to keep it submerged, then put muslin or cheesecloth over the top of the jar and seal it with a rubber band.

The cabbage needs five days to ferment at room temperature before it is transferred to the refrigerator, where it can be kept in an airtight container for up to six months.

SAFFRON YOGHURT

Making saffron yoghurt may seem like a bit of a luxury, but treating yourself is vital, and this is beautiful and has a delicate, delicious taste that makes a change from plain yoghurt.

small pinch of saffron strands
200g Greek yoghurt
2 tbsp lemon juice
1 tbsp extra virgin olive oil

194
kcal

Soak the saffron strands in about 3 tablespoons of just-boiled water for 10 minutes.

Mix together the yoghurt, saffron water (including the strands), lemon juice and olive oil. Transfer to an airtight container and keep in the fridge for up to 3 days.

INFUSED OILS

Nicole loves to add flavours to extra virgin olive oil and see what happens – a favourite is nori flakes. We also enjoy a combination of cardamom and black garlic, and one of the simplest is to add a few sprigs of rosemary to the bottle and wait a week or so for the flavour to infuse into the oil. These oils are perfect for adding a swirl of extra flavour to your soups.

STOCKS AND BROTHS

ROAST CHICKEN/ CHICKEN STOCK

This way of roasting the chicken is inspired by how the Chinese cook pork belly. It works a treat but do feel free to use your favourite recipe and then make your stock with the carcass. It's always useful to have some cooked chicken in the fridge for adding to soups.

MAKES 1 LITRE 130 kcal

1 medium chicken

1 lemon, cut in half

a few sprigs of rosemary

sea salt flakes, to season

1 onion, roughly chopped

1 leek, roughly chopped

2 bay leaves

1 tbsp tomato paste

1 small bunch fresh
   tarragon

Preheat the oven to 220°C/425°F/gas mark 7. Poke the chicken with a skewer vigorously all over to create small holes in the skin. Place the chicken in the sink and pour a kettle of boiling water over it (this is to help give a lovely crispy skin without overcooking the meat). Leave to drain, then pat dry and rub the lemon halves over the skin. Place the lemon halves in the cavity with the rosemary. Sprinkle the skin with the sea salt flakes.

Cook the chicken in the oven for 10 minutes, then lower the temperature to 140°C/275°F/ gas mark 1 and cook for 1–2 hours, depending on how large the chicken is.

To test if the chicken is done, pierce the thigh with a skewer and see if the liquid runs clear. If there is still blood, pop it back in the oven. When the chicken is cooked, switch off the heat and let it rest inside the oven for about half an hour.

To make the stock, preheat the oven to 140°C/275°F/gas mark 1. Pull all the meat off the chicken and set it aside – you can use it for a recipe or freeze it for another day. Put the bones into a large ovenproof casserole dish and cover with cold water. Bring the water to the boil on the hob, uncovered, then transfer the casserole to the oven to cook for 4 hours.

Return the casserole dish to the hob, leaving the oven on. Add the onion, leek, bay leaves and tomato paste. Bring to the boil, take it off the heat and put it back in the oven for an hour at the same temperature.

Add the tarragon to the stock after the hour, switch off the oven and leave to rest inside the oven.

Strain the stock through a sieve lined with muslin or cheesecloth, discarding all the solids. Transfer the stock to an airtight container once cool. Keeps for 3–4 days in the refrigerator, or can be frozen for 1 month.

SEAWEED BROTH

This makes a wonderful base for fish soups or an alternative to vegetable stock. It is also delicious by itself.

MAKES 1 LITRE 49 kcal

2 sheets kombu
1 celery stalk, roughly chopped
1 onion, roughly chopped
1 tsp black peppercorns
1 tsp capers

Add all the ingredients to a large pan and cover with 1.2 litres water. Bring to the boil, then leave to simmer for 45 minutes. Strain through a sieve lined with muslin or cheesecloth, discarding all the solids. Transfer the broth to an airtight container once cool. It will keep in the refrigerator for a week, or can be frozen for 1 month.

TURMERIC, GINGER AND LEMONGRASS BROTH

Turmeric is one of the most powerful natural anti-inflammatories known at present; it needs to be mixed with black pepper to be assimilated in the body for its greatest effect. Ginger root is also an anti-inflammatory as well as an antioxidant.

MAKES 1 LITRE 30 kcal

2 lemongrass
  stalks, bashed
1 tsp freshly grated
  turmeric
2 tsp freshly grated
  root ginger
juice of 1 lemon
freshly ground
  black pepper

Bring just over 1 litre of water to the boil in a pan with the lemongrass, then allow to simmer for 10 minutes. Add the turmeric, ginger, lemon juice and some black pepper and stir through for a couple of minutes, then take off the heat. Let the broth cool, then strain it through a sieve lined with muslin or cheesecloth, discarding all the solids.

Transfer the broth to an airtight container once cool. Drink the broth in small amounts either warmed or cool. It will keep in the refrigerator in an airtight container for a week, or can be frozen for 1 month.

BONE BROTH

The essence of all kitchens; this is the only red meat recipe included in the cleanse. We enjoy good-quality, organic red meat now and then, and in this broth form it is easy to absorb all the nutrients.

MAKES 1 LITRE 220 kcal

1kg veal or beef
   marrow bones
500g beef scraps
500g chicken wings
1 onion, quartered
1 leek, roughly chopped
1 celery stalk, roughly
   chopped
1 garlic clove

Preheat the oven to 220°C/425°F/gas mark 7. Place the bones and beef scraps in a roasting tin and cook in the oven for 2 hours, until well coloured. Transfer the bones and scraps to a large pot with the remaining ingredients and about 2 litres of water, bring to the boil and gently simmer on a very low heat for up to 8 hours, scooping off any fat that comes to the surface (don't put it down the sink as it will solidify and block the drain).

Strain the stock through a sieve lined with muslin or cheesecloth, discarding all the solids. Transfer the stock to an airtight container once cool. It will keep in the refrigerator for a week, or can be frozen for 1 month.

VEGETABLE STOCK

This makes quite a delicate, aromatic white vegetable stock; perfect for the cleanse recipes.

MAKES 1 LITRE 78 kcal

1 leek, roughly chopped

1 white onion, roughly chopped

¼ celeriac, roughly chopped

1 celery, roughly chopped

1 fennel, roughly chopped

6 garlic cloves, bashed

1 tsp coriander seeds

sea salt flakes

a handful of soft herbs – such as dill, coriander, tarragon

Add all the chopped vegetables to a large pot, along with the garlic, coriander seeds and a little salt and cover with about 1.2 litres of water. Bring to the boil, then reduce the heat to a good simmer and cook for 45 minutes until all the vegetables have softened. Switch off the heat and add your preferred soft herbs, then leave to rest for an hour or so before straining through a sieve lined with muslin or cheesecloth, discarding all the solids.

Transfer the stock to an airtight container once cool. It will keep in the refrigerator for a week, or can be frozen for 1 month.

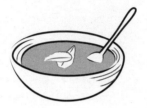

CHAPTER 8:
BEYOND THE CLEANSE

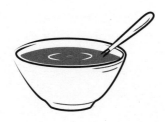

We hope that our soup cleanses inspire you to include more soups in your day-to-day diet and that they help you to get into or back into the habit of cooking easy and delicious healthy recipes from scratch.

We are far from saintly ourselves, so we also need to remind ourselves every now and then of a few simple principles for happy and healthy living. We always feel at our best when we are in balance with ourselves and our bodies, exercising regularly (if never obsessively), eating natural foods and enjoying life.

TIPS FOR LIFE BEYOND THE CLEANSE

HEALTHY EATING

After the cleanse, try to keep your kitchen tidy and topped up with healthy ingredients. Always have a few different grains such as quinoa, buckwheat, barley and rice, along with lentils, and plenty of spices and seeds to hand, for scattering over soups to add a bit of crunch.

Try not to leave spices lingering too long at the back of a cupboard – experiment with them by making different recipes. We usually have a container of tofu in the fridge that is marinating in various spices, we just open up the drawer and see what looks good – sumac and za'atar, nori flakes and sesame, turmeric and cumin.

Plan your meals for the week ahead, looking at what you already have and then adding your fresh ingredients. Batch cooking on Sunday is such a great way to set up a healthy week of eating, from soups for your lunches or a lovely stew that will keep you going early on in the week with different vegetables.

Keep making stock, especially chicken and vegetable. It's the basis of so many great dishes and you have delicious roast chicken to enjoy, too.

Try to eat fresh fish at least once or twice a week. Cold-water oily fish such as salmon, mackerel, sardines and anchovies are particularly good as they are packed with healthy fats.

Be adventurous while also knowing you can fall back on a growing list of healthy favourites. People often tell us that our lemon, chicken and mint soup has become one of their household staples (it is good!).

Don't fall back into old habits of being on the computer or watching television while eating. Keep meal times for eating or for sharing.

Watch out for your portion sizes, it's easy for them to creep up and being mindful of them is a great way to keep your diet in balance.

Keep up with drinking plenty of water and herbal teas; the best thing is to experiment and find your favourites as there are so many different teas to choose from.

Try not to become too controlling about food. Don't feel guilty for having a cake. Relax and enjoy it. It's amazing how well the digestive system responds in kind.

HEALTHY LIVING

Always find ways to be as active as possible throughout the day. If you work in an office, for example, go for a walk at lunchtime or walk or cycle some of the way to work and back home. Make a conscious effort to get up from your desk every couple of hours to stretch your legs and clear your mind.

Find an exercise that you really enjoy. It might be a class once or twice a week such as kettle bells, Zumba or spinning. You might love CrossFit, or swimming, cycling or running. If you love yoga, go for it. There are so many choices nowadays that even if you didn't love the sports on offer while at school, there's bound to be something that works for you.

Start small when making changes. It's amazing how well the running apps work, simply adding a couple of minutes each day until suddenly you're up to 5k or 10k. The same goes for creating any kind of healthy habit – long-term changes come from taking one small step at a time.

Continue to take time out for yourself beyond the cleanse. Your mind and your body are so incredible, why not treat them and take care of them, whether through quiet contemplation in the morning or evening, booking a regular massage appointment or taking up a meditation class.

Forgive us for sounding a little 'woo woo' but for us, gratitude is a big part of living healthily and in balance. The more we appreciate everything in our lives, the better we feel about ourselves and naturally want to take care of our bodies.

Be curious about yourself, how you feel and what you need today to feel nourished.

NUTRITIONAL INFORMATION

THE SOUPS

RESOLVE

Avocado, lemon, turmeric and cayenne
Per serving: 163 calories;
2g protein; 15g total fat; 9g
saturated fat; 7g carbohydrate;
4g fibre; 290mg sodium

Corn, kale and avocado
Per serving: 230 calories;
7g protein; 17g total fat;
10g saturated fat;
18g carbohydrate; 13g fibre;
51mg sodium

Balti-spiced cauliflower
Per serving: 214 calories;
6g protein; 15g total fat;
2g saturated fat;
19g carbohydrate; 7g fibre; |
80mg sodium

Beetroot, coconut and salmon
Per serving: 307 calories;
18g protein; 15g total fat;
12g saturated fat;
29g carbohydrate; 6g fibre;
219mg sodium

Chicken soup for the cleansed soul
Per serving: 286 calories;
28g protein; 16g total fat;
3g saturated fat; 8g carbohydrate;
3g fibre; 241mg sodium

Curried parsnip and apple
Per serving: 277 calories;
2g protein; 19g total fat;
11g saturated fat;
24g carbohydrate; 8g fibre;
52mg sodium

Green gazpacho
Per serving: 199 calories;
5g protein; 15g total fat;
3g saturated fat;
13g carbohydrate; 6g fibre;
30mg sodium

Hot cucumber with salmon
Per serving: 275 calories;
24g protein; 10g total fat;
3g saturated fat; 18g
carbohydrate; 3g fibre;
802mg sodium

Hot cucumber with barley
Per serving: 206 calories;
6g protein; 3g total fat;
2g saturated fat;
37g carbohydrate; 7g fibre;
561mg sodium

Leek, fennel and celery with red lentils

Per serving: 237 calories;
11g protein; 8g total fat;
1g saturated fat;
32g carbohydrate; 12g fibre;
179mg sodium

Spiced cod with samphire

Per serving: 349 calories;
28g protein; 18g total fat;
13g saturated fat;
18g carbohydrate; 5g fibre;
596mg sodium

Salmon poached in lemongrass tea

Per serving: 309 calories;
31g protein; 20g total fat;
5g saturated fat; 2g carbohydrate;
1g fibre; 115mg sodium

Summer chicken

Per serving: 268 calories;
38g protein; 6g total fat;
3g saturated fat; 14g
carbohydrate; 5g fibre;
37mg sodium

Wild garlic, baby spinach and olive

Per serving: 211 calories;
4g protein; 15g total fat;
2g saturated fat;
14g carbohydrate; 2g fibre;
450mg sodium

REBALANCE

Asparagus mimosa

Per serving: 241 calories;
14g protein; 14g total fat;
3g saturated fat;
15g carbohydrate; 3g fibre;
573mg sodium

Chicken and courgette Thai noodle soup

Per serving: 383 calories;
33g protein; 21g total fat;
16g saturated fat;
6g carbohydrate; 1g fibre;
170mg sodium

Coconut chicken with turmeric and kale

Per serving: 378 calories;
24g protein; 22g total fat;
13g saturated fat;
26g carbohydrate; 6g fibre;
108mg sodium

Courgette, lemon and thyme

Per serving: 188 calories;
5g protein; 18g total fat;
3g saturated fat; 4g carbohydrate;
2g fibre; 17mg sodium

Five-spice tofu

Per serving: 146 calories;
15g protein; 8g total fat;
1g saturated fat; 6g carbohydrate;
3g fibre; 426mg sodium

Harissa cauliflower and corn

Per serving: 239 calories;
9g protein; 10g total fat;
1g saturated fat;
30g carbohydrate; 12g fibre;
158mg sodium

Horseradish and lemony squash

Per serving: 316 calories;
6g protein; 20g total fat;
3g saturated fat; 32g
carbohydrate; 7g fibre;
73mg sodium

Kitchari

Per serving: 219 calories;
6g protein; 17g total fat;
13g saturated fat; 16g
carbohydrate; 5g fibre;
14mg sodium

Lemon, chicken and mint

Per serving: 174 calories;
20g protein; 8g total fat;
2g saturated fat; 8g carbohydrate;
2g fibre; 126mg sodium

Pea and preserved lemon

Per serving: 134 calories;
11g protein; 3g total fat;
1g saturated fat; 21g carbohydrate;
5g fibre; 550mg sodium

Roasted cherry tomato and lemon soup with salsa

Per serving: 133 calories;
2g protein; 8g total fat;
1g saturated fat; 13g carbohydrate;
4g fibre; 52mg sodium

Saffron broth with fish

Per serving: 133 calories;
24g protein; 1g total fat;
0.2g saturated fat;
6g carbohydrate; 3g fibre;
274mg sodium

Sichuan pepper and chicken

Per serving: 268 calories;
21g protein; 15g total fat;
4g saturated fat; 8g carbohydrate;
4g fibre; 877mg sodium

Smoked aubergine and kefir

Per serving: 135 calories;
4g protein; 8g total fat;
2g saturated fat; 13g carbohydrate;
4g fibre; 31mg sodium

Hot smoked mushroom

Per serving: 100 calories;
4g protein; 8g total fat;
6g saturated fat;
6g total carbohydrate; 2g fibre;
50mg sodium

Spinach and spiced onion

Per serving: 180 calories;
5g protein; 9g total fat;
6g saturated fat;
18g carbohydrate; 6g fibre;
87mg sodium

Spring chicken

Per serving: 302 calories;
35g protein; 13g total fat;
4g saturated fat; 7g carbohydrate;
3g fibre; 57mg sodium

Tofu sea spaghetti miso

Per serving: 340 calories;
19g protein; 24g total fat;
4g saturated fat;
13g carbohydrate; 8g fibre;
1008mg sodium

Smoked tofu, tomato and broccoli

Per serving: 111 calories;
6g protein; 5g total fat;
1g saturated fat;
10g carbohydrate; 4g fibre;
134mg sodium

RESTORE

Autumn chicken

Per serving: 266 calories;
33g protein; 12g total fat;
4g saturated fat; 3g carbohydrate;
2g fibre; 25mg sodium

Buckwheat broth

Per serving: 295 calories;
11g protein; 9g total fat;
6g saturated fat;
45g carbohydrate; 8g fibre;
1216mg sodium

Butternut squash and sage

Per serving: 309 calories;
6g protein; 15g total fat;
2g saturated fat;
45g carbohydrate; 13g fibre;
39mg sodium

Cardamom coconut barley

Per serving: 386 calories;
13g protein; 27g total fat;
19g saturated fat;
23g carbohydrate; 3g fibre;
116mg sodium

Carrot, cumin and miso soup with grain salad

Per serving: 179 calories;
3g protein; 8g total fat;
6g saturated fat;
27g carbohydrate; 8g fibre;
231mg sodium

For the salad

Per serving: 115 calories;
5g protein; 1g total fat;
0g saturated fat;
22g carbohydrate; 4g fibre;
10mg sodium

Carrot, ginger and tangerine

Per serving: 146 calories;
2g protein; 8g total fat;
1g saturated fat; 19g carbohydrate;
5g fibre; 186mg sodium

Celeriac and umami mustard

Per serving: 199 calories;
3g protein; 16g total fat;
2g saturated fat;
18g carbohydrate; 9g fibre;
186mg sodium

Chicken congee

Per serving: 388 calories;
34g protein; 13g total fat;
3g saturated fat;
29g carbohydrate; 2g dietary
fibre; 1115mg sodium

Cinnamon pumpkin

Per serving: 116 calories;
2g protein; 7g total fat;
1g saturated fat; 9g carbohydrate;
4g fibre; 43mg sodium

Cod laksa

Per serving: 207 calories;
29g protein; 10g total fat;
3g saturated fat;
9g carbohydrate; 2g fibre;
269mg sodium

Cumin-roasted sweet potato with onion and pomegranate molasses

Per serving: 295 calories;
3g protein; 15g total fat;
2g saturated fat;
38g carbohydrate; 3g fibre;
110mg sodium

Ginger carrot with spiced coconut yoghurt

Per serving: 384 calories;
6g protein; 24g total fat;
9g saturated fat;
36g carbohydrate; 11g fibre;
262mg sodium

Jerusalem artichoke and fennel

Per serving: 314 calories;
7g protein; 18g total fat;
2g saturated fat;
34g carbohydrate; 5g fibre;
67mg sodium

Lentils, seasonal greens and ginger carrot coleslaw

Per serving: 343 calories;
18g protein; 13g total fat;
3g saturated fat;
29g carbohydrate; 10g fibre;
50mg sodium

Magic soup

Per serving: 343 calories;
19g protein; 12g total fat;
7g saturated fat; 41g carbohydrate;
16g fibre; 76mg sodium

Roasted buckwheat with achari spices and exotic mushrooms

Per serving: 305 calories;
7g protein; 16g total fat;
8g saturated fat;
35g carbohydrate; 7g fibre;
93mg sodium

Sprouted soup

Per serving: 245 calories;
7g protein; 16g total fat;
3g saturated fat;
19g carbohydrate; 5g fibre;
23mg sodium

White kimchi

Per serving: 118 calories;
8g protein; 6g fat; 2g saturated fat;
3g carbohydrate; 2g fibre;
2800mg sodium

RENEW

Barley bone broth
Per serving: 284 calories;
6g protein; 12g total fat;
2g saturated fat;
35g carbohydrate; 6g fibre;
87mg sodium

Beetroot and caraway
Per serving: 136 calories;
6g protein; 1g total fat;
1g saturated fat;
24g carbohydrate; 5g fibre;
112mg sodium

Cauliflower, garlic and walnut crumb
Per serving: 256 calories;
9g protein; 12g total fat;
1g saturated fat; 32g carbohydrate;
11g fibre; 236mg sodium

Chicken and nettle tops
Per serving: 274 calories;
44g protein; 5g total fat;
2g saturated fat; 11g carbohydrate;
3g fibre; 1939mg sodium

Fennel-crusted salmon with ginger Chinese cabbage
Per serving: 311 calories;
31g protein; 15g total fat;
4g saturated fat;
10g carbohydrate; 3g fibre;
140mg sodium

Harissa broth with aubergine and quinoa
Per serving: 194 calories;
4g protein; 12g total fat;
2g saturated fat; 16g carbohydrate;
4g fibre; 276mg sodium

Green pho
Per serving: 77 calories;
5g protein; 1g total fat;
0g saturated fat; 9g carbohydrate;
4g fibre; 106mg sodium

Mussels and leek
Per serving: 372 calories;
32g protein; 13g total fat;
6g saturated fat;
25g carbohydrate; 3g fibre;
731mg sodium

Raw soup
Per serving: 194 calories;
4g protein; 12g total fat;
3g saturated fat; 11g carbohydrate;
6g fibre; 13mg sodium

Crab, fennel and turmeric congee
Per serving: 316 calories;
19g protein; 13g total fat;
3g saturated fat;
28g carbohydrate; 1g fibre;
120mg sodium

Red lentil and tamarind
Per serving: 204 calories;
8g protein; 3g total fat;
1g saturated fat;
35g carbohydrate; 8g fibre;
130mg sodium

Roast chickpea
Per serving: 188 calories;
1g protein; 1g total fat;
1g saturated fat; 13g carbohydrate;
2g fibre; 11mg sodium

Sesame chicken
Per serving: 362 calories;
30g protein; 12g total fat;
3g saturated fat; 32g carbohydrate;
3g fibre; 851mg sodium

Sopa de quinoa
Per serving: 381 calories;
6g protein; 33g total fat;
5g saturated fat;
18g carbohydrate; 6g fibre;
102mg sodium

Squash and almond butter
Per serving: 376 calories;
9g protein; 17g total fat;
2g saturated fat; 51g carbohydrate;
11g fibre; 19mg sodium

Watercress, flax and tofu
Per serving: 248 calories;
14g protein; 17g total fat; 3g
saturated fat; 10g carbohydrate;
4g fibre; 347mg sodium

Wild rice, edamame and rainbow chard
Per serving: 165 calories;
7g protein; 4g fat; 1g saturated fat;
24g carbohydrate; 4g fibre;
235mg sodium

Winter chicken
Per serving: 336 calories;
36g protein; 18g total fat;
5g saturated fat; 5g carbohydrate;
2g fibre; 42mg sodium

SOUP JARS

Kimchi miso tofu
Per serving: 380 calories;
16g protein; 5g total fat;
1g saturated fat; 66g
carbohydrate; 5g fibre; 1271mg
sodium

Coconut prawn
Per serving: 391 calories;
23g protein; 3g total fat;
1g saturated fat; 71g carbohydrate;
5g fibre; 670mg sodium

Shiitake seaweed miso
Per serving: 178 calories;
13g protein; 6g total fat;
1g saturated fat; 21g carbohydrate;
18g fibre; 217mg sodium

Chicken and baby kale laksa
Per serving: 370 calories;
29g protein; 3g total fat;
1g saturated fat; 38g
carbohydrate; 2g fibre;
213mg sodium

CLEANSE-ENHANCING RECIPES

BREAKFAST

Overnight oats
Per serving: 221 calories;
8g protein; 8g total fat;
2g saturated fat; 30g
carbohydrate; 8g fibre;
114mg sodium

Clove-spiced apple
Per serving: 165 calories;
2g protein; 8g total fat;
4g saturated fat; 26g
carbohydrate; 5g fibre;
2mg sodium

Bircher
Per serving: 152 calories;
3g protein; 5g total fat; 1g
saturated fat; 27g carbohydrate;
5g fibre; 2mg sodium

Berry compote
Per serving: 59 calories;
0g protein; 0g fat;
14g carbohydrate; 1g fibre;
7mg sodium

Egg drop soup with nori
Per serving: 260 calories;
17g protein; 15g total fat;
3g saturated fat; 15g carbohydrate;
4g fibre; 1771mg sodium

Miso breakfast broth
Per serving: 148 calories;
9g protein; 5g total fat; 1g
saturated fat; 18g carbohydrate;
6g fibre; 274mg sodium

SMOOTHIES

Berry kefir booster
Per serving: 146 calories;
6g protein; 2g total fat;
1g saturated fat;
28g carbohydrate; 4g fibre;
99mg sodium

Almond chia
Per serving: 312 calories;
8g protein; 18g total fat;
6g saturated fat; 32g
carbohydrate; 8g fibre;
61mg sodium

Avocado nuts
Per serving: 271 calories;
6g protein; 21g total fat;
2g saturated fat; 17g carbohydrate;
7g fibre; 231mg sodium

SNACKS

Nourish bites
Per bite: 150 calories;
3g protein; 10g total fat;
5g saturated fat; 13g carbohydrate;
3g fibre; 15mg sodium

Kale crisps
Per 25g serving: 56 calories;
2g protein; 5g total fat;
1g saturated fat; 2g carbohydrate;
1g fibre; 82mg sodium

Turmeric and black pepper oatcakes
Per oatcake: 51 calories;
1g protein; 2g total fat;
1g saturated fat; 8g carbohydrate;
1g fibre; 29mg sodium

PASTES, CHUTNEYS AND MAKE-AHEAD GARNISHES

Laksa paste
Per tablespoon serving:
26 calories; 0.5g protein; 2g fat;
0g saturated fat; 2g carbohydrate;
0.5g fibre; 3mg sodium

Thai paste
Per tablespoon serving:
16 calories; 1g protein; 0g total fat;
4g carbohydrate; 1g fibre;
8mg sodium

Celeriac and umami mustard paste
Per teaspoon serving:
14 calories; 0g protein;
0.5g total fat; 0g saturated fat;
1g carbohydrate; 0g fibre;
7mg sodium

Cleanse spice mix
Per teaspoon serving:
12 calories; 1g protein; 1g total fat;
0g saturated fat; 1g carbohydrate;
1g fibre; 2mg sodium

Cleanse dukkah
Per teaspoon serving:
17 calories; 1g protein;
1.4g total fat; 0g saturated fat;
0.5g carbohydrates; 0g fibre;
0mg sodium

Kimchi
Per 100g: 42 calories; 2g protein;
0.2g fat; 7g carbohydrate; 3g fibre;
2810mg sodium

Saffron yoghurt
Per 100g: 194 calories; 5g protein;
17 g total fat; 7g saturated fat;
8g carbohydrate; 0g fibre;
91mg sodium

STOCKS AND BROTHS

Roast chicken/Chicken stock
Per litre: 130 calories; 16g protein;
5g total fat; 1g saturated fat;
4g carbohydrate; 5g fibre;
442mg sodium

Seaweed broth
Per litre: 49 calories; 2g protein;
1g total fat; 0.5g saturated fat;
8g carbohydrate; 2g fibre;
648mg sodium

Turmeric, ginger and lemongrass broth
Per litre: 30 calories; 1g protein;
0g fat; 8g carbohydrate; 1g fibre;
8mg sodium

Bone broth
Per litre: 220 calories; 32g protein;
5g total fat; 1g saturated fat;
9g carbohydrate; 5g fibre;
169mg sodium

Vegetable stock
Per litre: 78 calories; 1g protein;
1g fat; 0g saturated fat;
11g carbohydrate; 2g fibre;
368 mg sodium

Nicole Pisani was a senior chef at Nopi in Soho, London, for Yotam Ottolenghi and before that worked with Anna Hansen at The Modern Pantry. She is currently the chef for Gayhurst Primary School in Hackney, and works closely with Henry Dimbleby and the School Food Plan. Nicole has always had a passion for inspiring people to eat well and cook for themselves. She will introduce you to ingredients, techniques and flavour combinations that you'll want to share with everyone you know!

'I can't help but share food and, I hope, a little inspiration for adventures in your own kitchen.'

Kate Adams is a writer with a passion for food, health and happiness. She was the health publisher for Penguin Books, before changing her life for the better, taking her health into her own hands and losing two and half stone in the process. Kate now runs www.flattummyclub.co.uk and works with an eclectic mix of health experts, entrepreneurs and Buddhist lamas.

'I believe in making it easier for real people to live well, to eat simply and deliciously, to feel a sense of balance in themselves and their bodies, and to be happy.'

Nicole and Kate's first cookbook together was *Magic Soup*, published by Orion.

For more delicious recipes and inspiration visit the website **www.foodforhappiness.co.uk** or the Twitter page **@happyfoodco** and **#ultimatesoupcleanse**.

ACKNOWLEDGEMENTS

Thank you for buying this book and for cooking our recipes – we hope you've enjoyed them!

Thank you to the team at Orion, especially Tamsin, Amanda and Helen, and to Clare Hulton. Thanks also to Victoria Wells for her invaluable nutritional advice.

Thanks as ever to our friend and talented photographer Regula Ysewijn.

And to our mentors and teachers, without whom we'd never have been able to create so many soups!

INDEX

For more delicious recipes by
Nicole Pisani and Kate Adams
look out for
Magic Soup, available now from
all good bookshops and online.

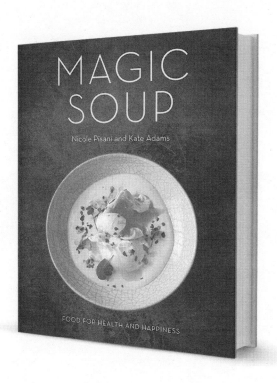

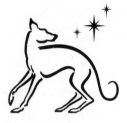